MY STORY

Have you heard of a term called kintsugi? It is the traditional Japanese art of using precious metal, or lacquer dusted with precious metal, to repair broken pottery, putting together the broken pieces, making it more beautiful and stronger. To me, kintsugi is the art of embracing our brokenness, or our wounds, and becoming stronger. I have been hammered several times by situations and people in my life, which shattered me into pieces. During earth-shattering moments in my life, I gained strength from my gratitude jar. I developed an attitude of gratitude and it helped me to focus on my blessings and stay grounded. Over the period, I learned the art of forgiveness, patience, unconditional love, and unconditional acceptance, which is my precious metal, and these have helped me heal my wounds.

Hence now I strive to pay it forward and spread the hope so that you can heal and live life to the fullest. You are not alone in this journey, as I have got your back. The attitude of gratitude will help you stay positive and focused on your blessings. When you count your blessings, you will maintain your sanity during hard times and attract more blessings in your life.

- Kruti Thakore
Radiant Confidence

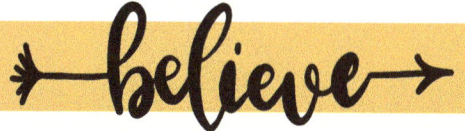

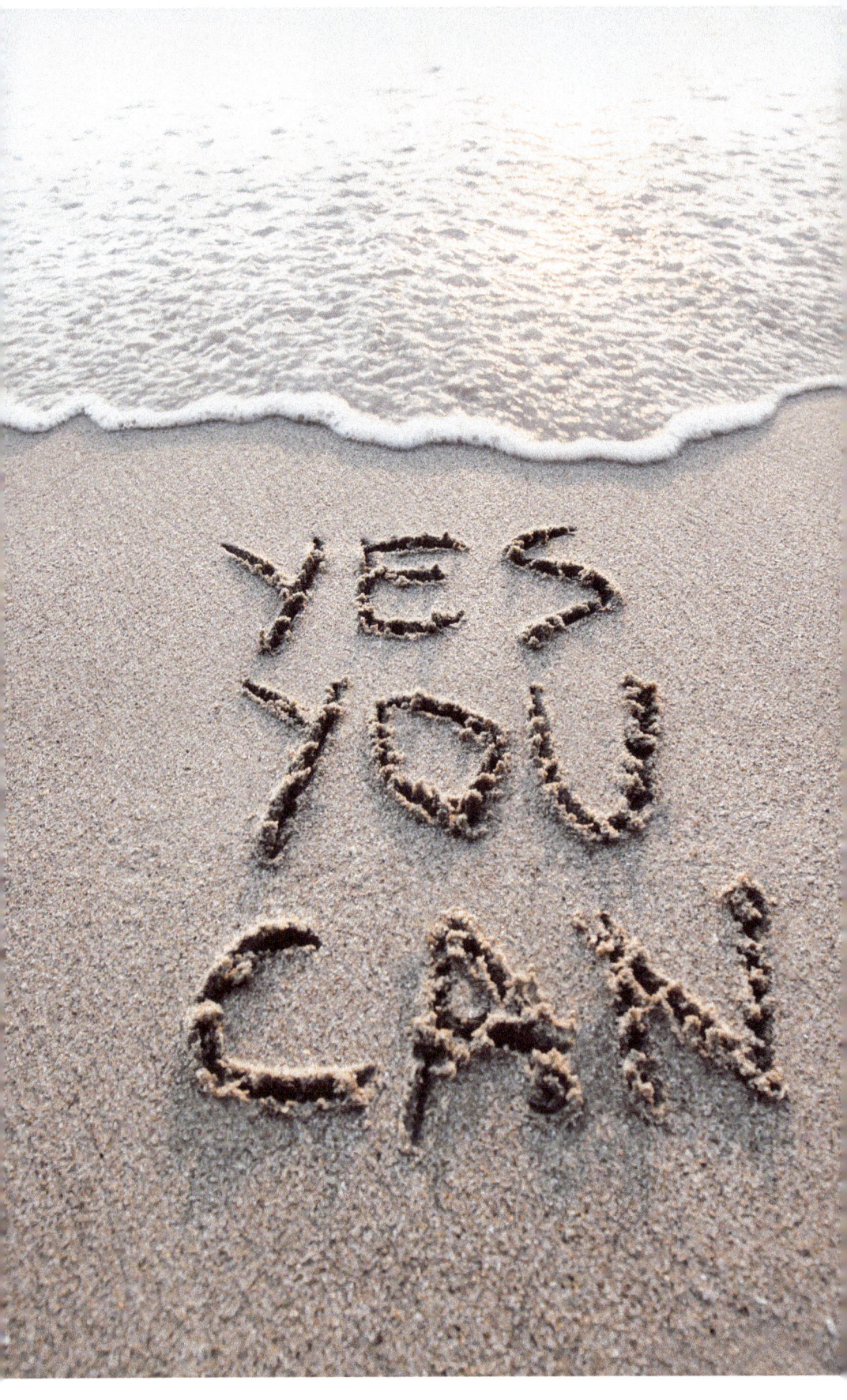

AN ATTITUDE OF GRATITUDE HELPS US BE MORE RESILIENT

I AM GRATEFUL FOR...

hope

INSPIRE Someone TODAY

AN ATTITUDE OF GRATITUDE GIVES EMOTIONAL STABILITY

I AM GRATEFUL FOR...

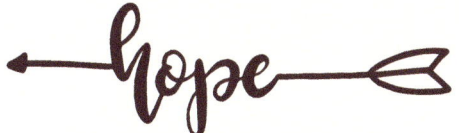

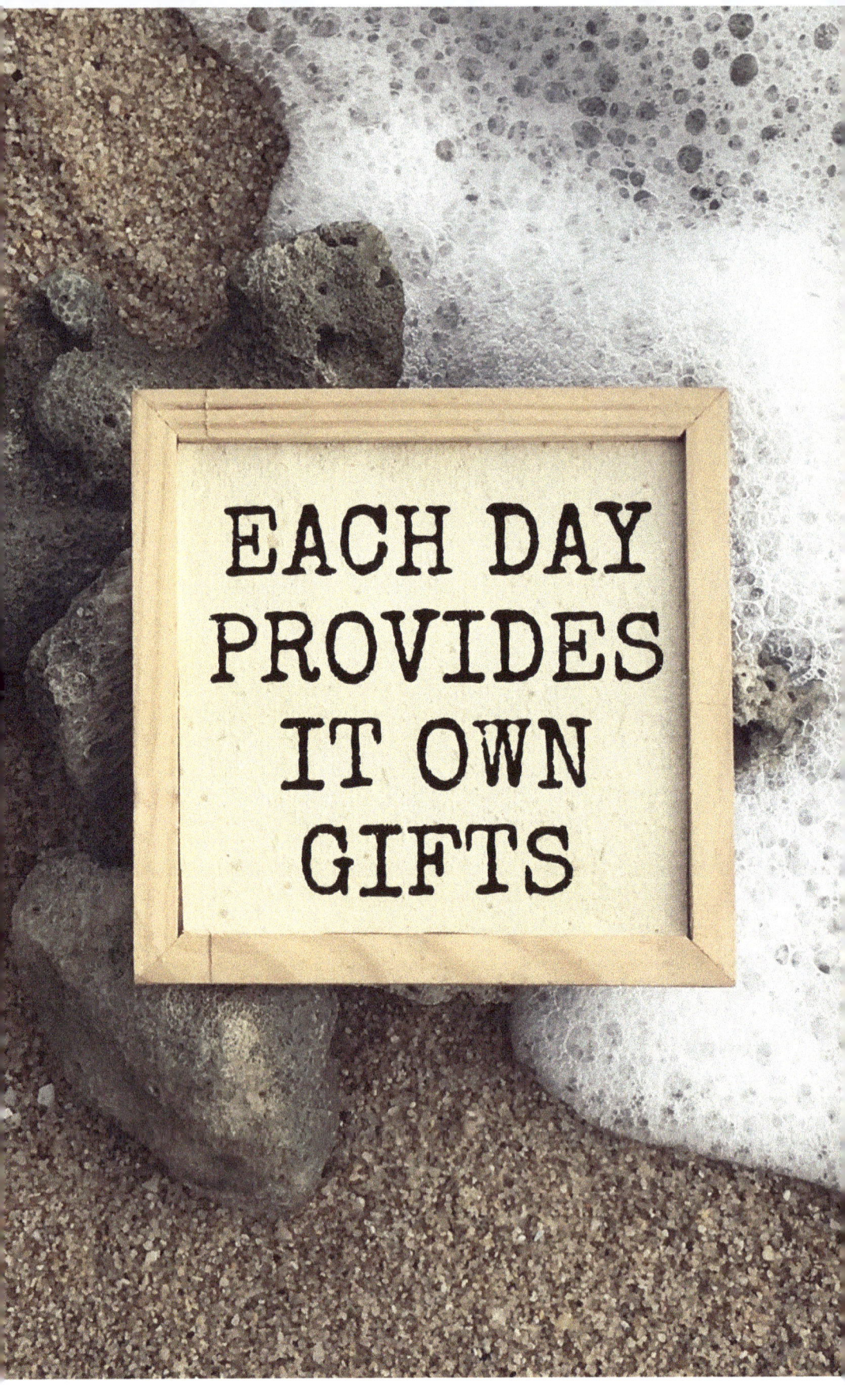

AN ATTITUDE OF GRATITUDE MAKES US HAPPIER BECAUSE IT IS DIFFICULT TO BE SAD WHEN WE ARE GRATEFUL.

I AM GRATEFUL FOR...

hope

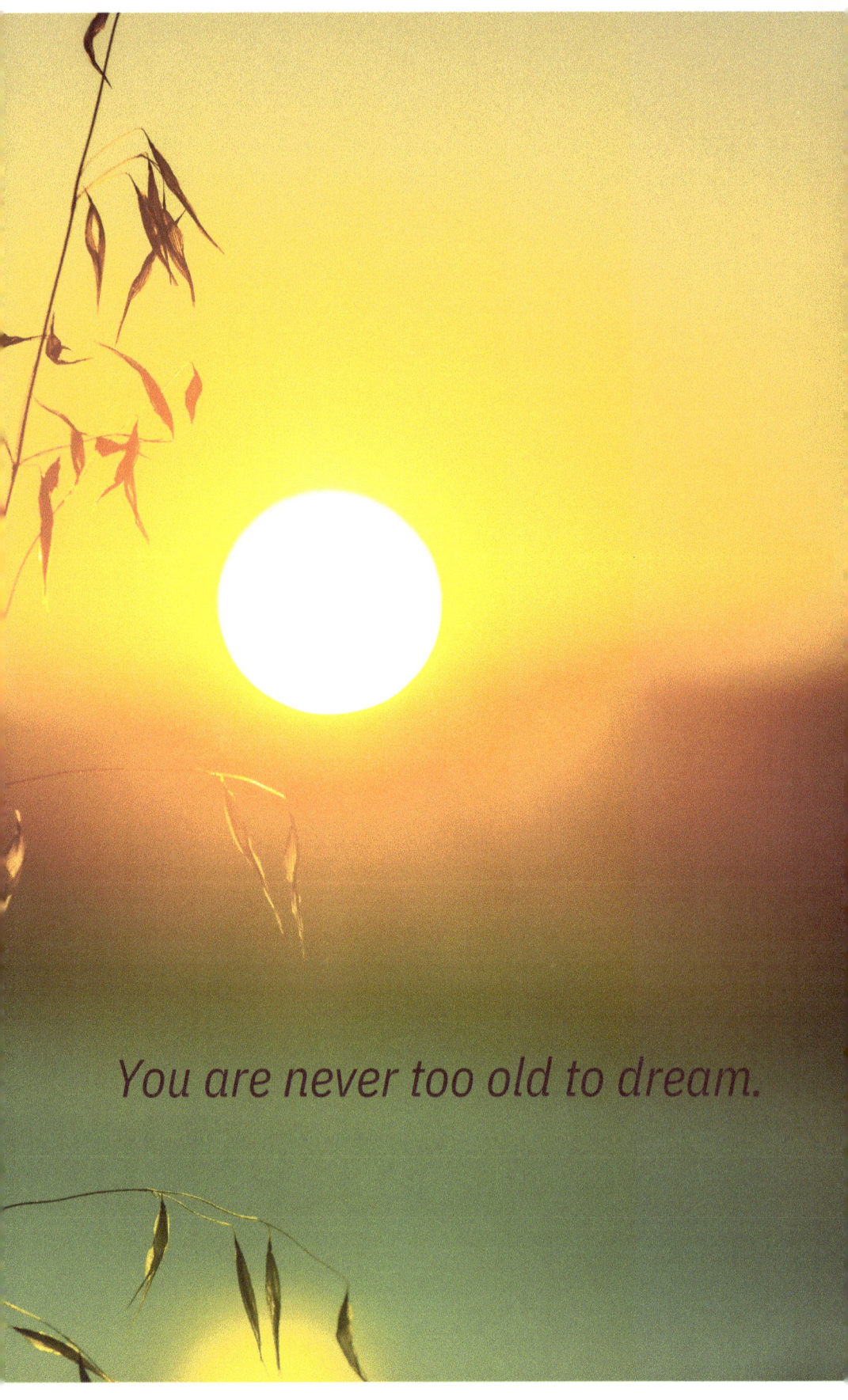

WHEN I STARTED COUNTING MY BLESSINGS, IT CHANGED MY LIFE FOR THE BETTER.

I AM GRATEFUL FOR...

hope

THE BEST VIEW COMES AFTER THE HARDEST CLIMB

AN ATTITUDE OF GRATITUDE IMPROVES RELATIONSHIPS AS IT KEEPS US FOCUSED ON THE POSITIVE

I AM GRATEFUL FOR...

hope

**BE STRONGER
THAN YOUR
EXCUSES**

GRATITUDE -> OPTIMISM -> AN EXTRA FEW MONTHS OR YEARS ON EARTH.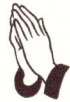

I AM GRATEFUL FOR...

BE POSITIVE, PATIENT AND PERSISTENT.

GRATITUDE HELPS US BOUNCE BACK FASTER.

I AM GRATEFUL FOR...

hope

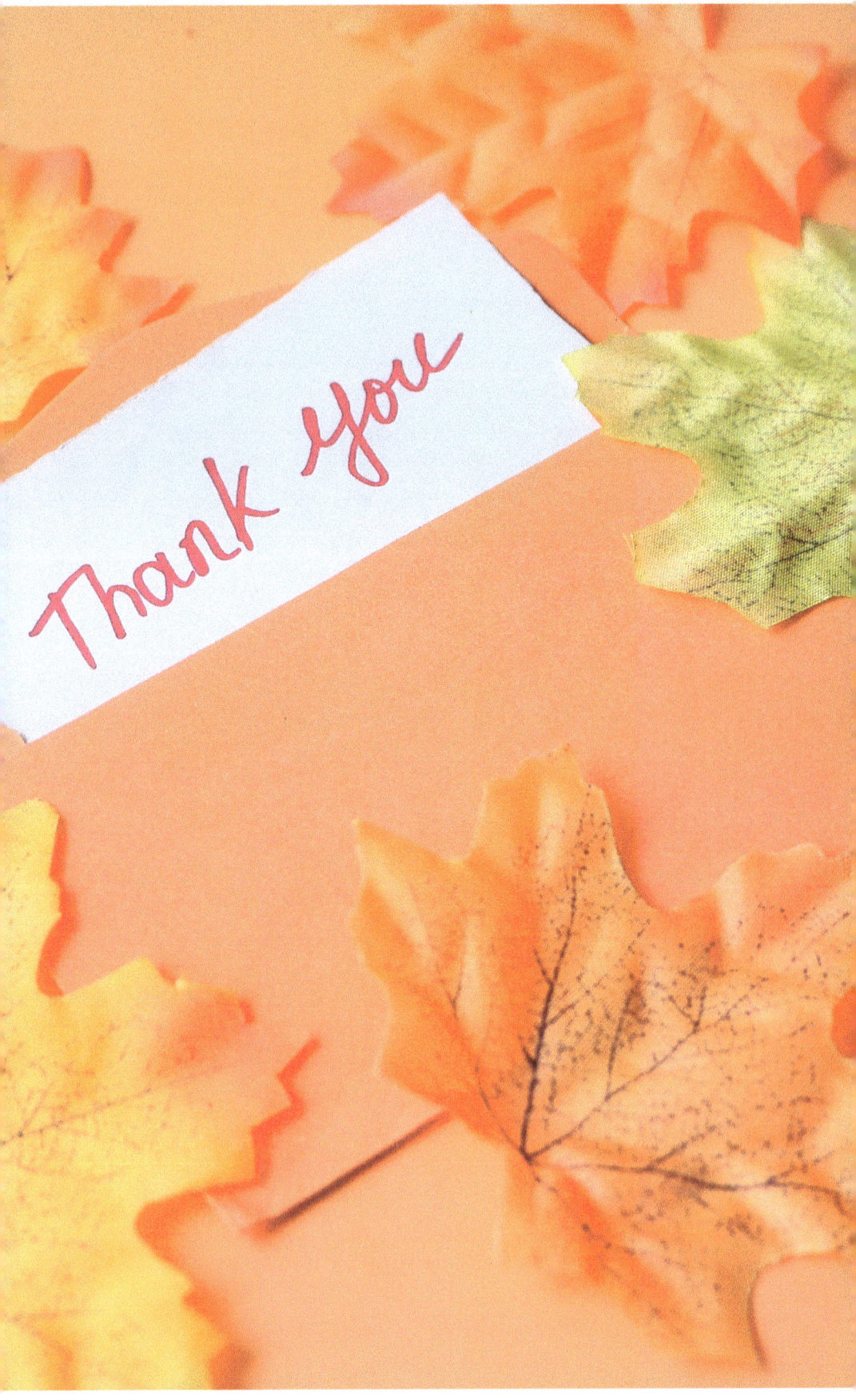

TODAY MORNING I OPENED THE TWO BEST GIFTS ON THIS PLANET; MY EYES.

I AM GRATEFUL FOR...

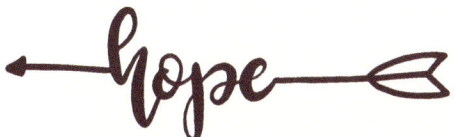

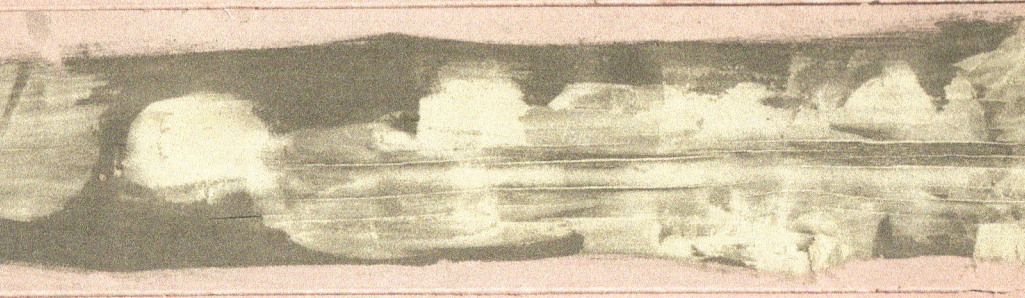

AN ATTITUDE OF GRATITUDE TRAINS OUR MINDS TO SEE GOOD IN EVERY SITUATION.

TODAY I AM GRATEFUL FOR...

hope

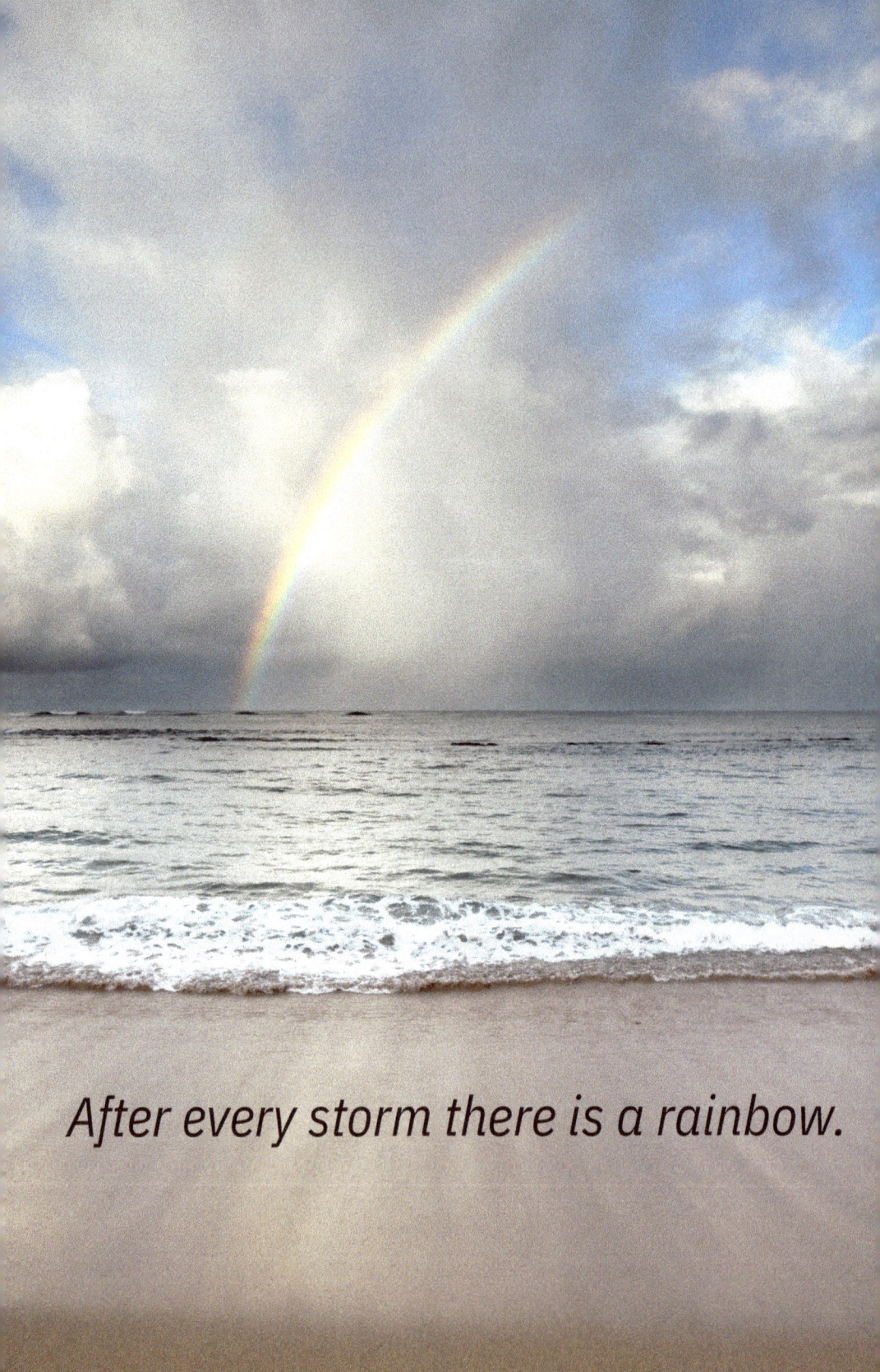

COUNT YOUR BLESSINGS AND YOU SHALL RECEIVE MORE BLESSINGS TO COUNT.

I AM GRATEFUL FOR...

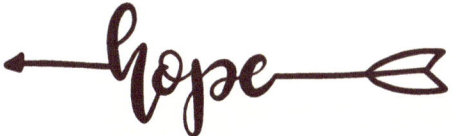

never lose HOPE.

AN ATTITUDE OF GRATITUDE WILL LOWER YOUR STRESS LEVELS.

I AM GRATEFUL FOR...

hope

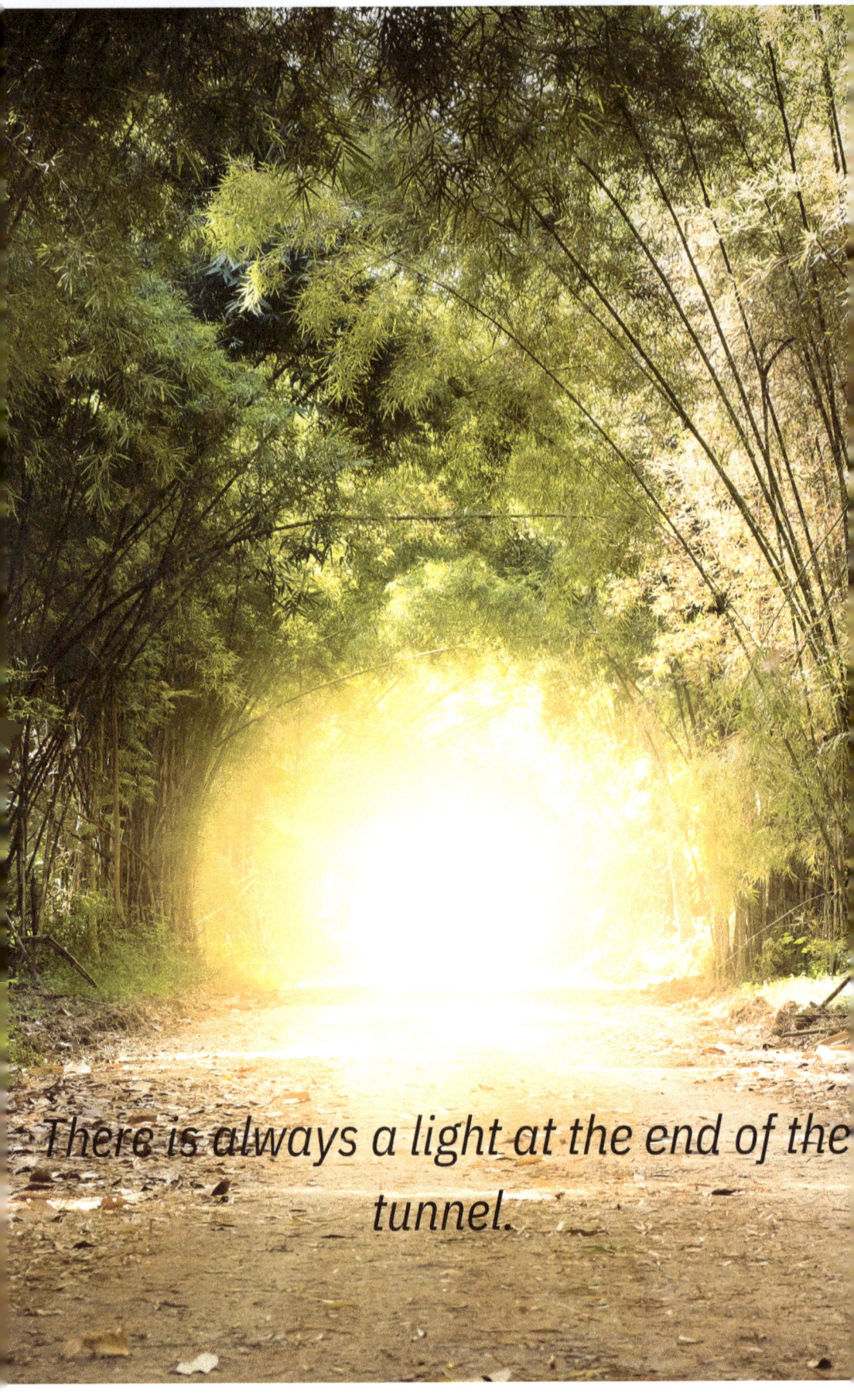

GRATITUDE HELPS YOU CHANGE YOUR PERSPECTIVE.

I AM GRATEFUL FOR...

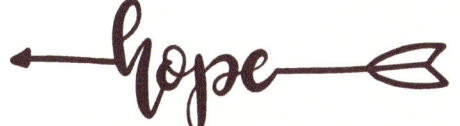

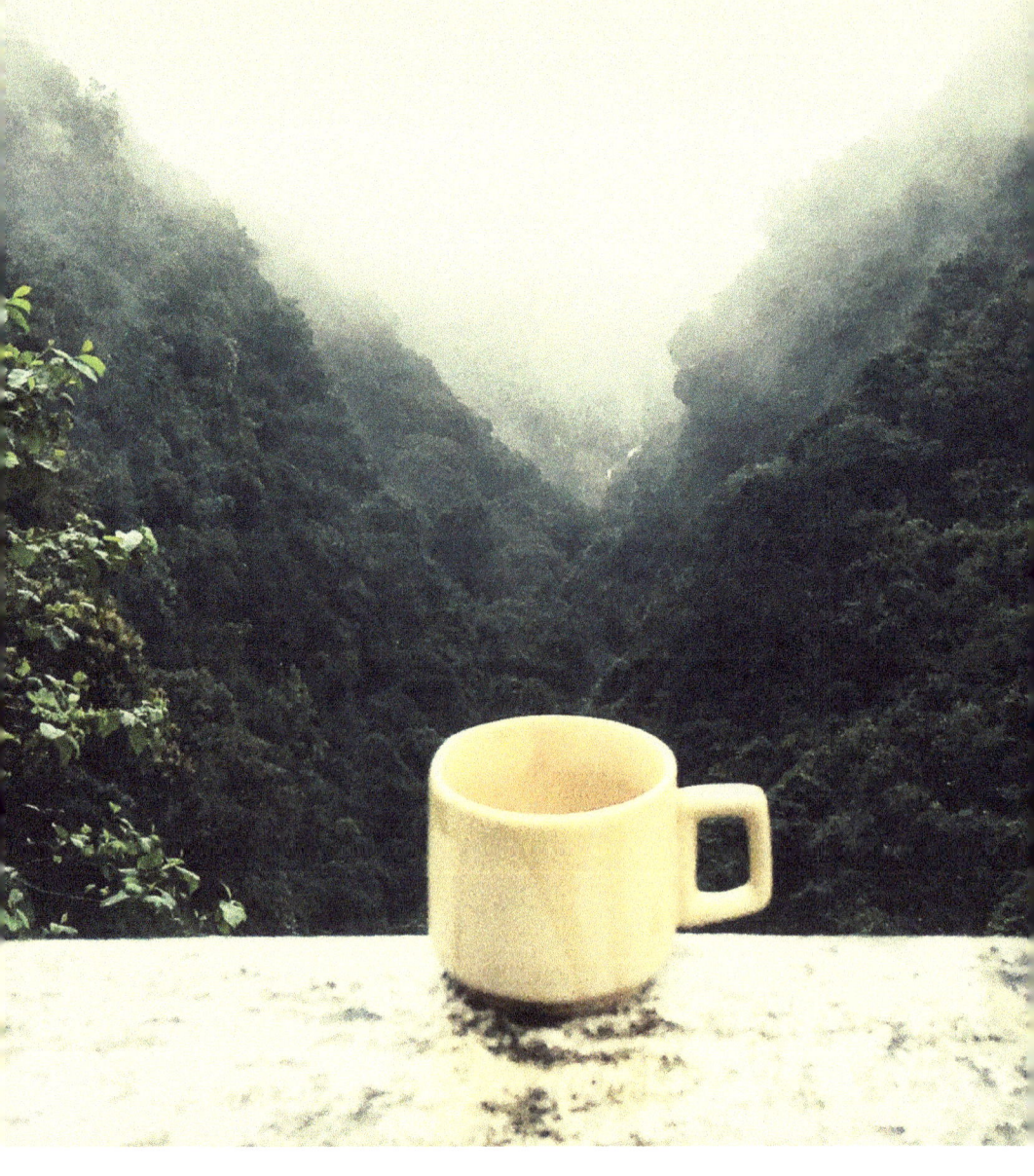

> Every morning when I open my curtains for that first look at the day, no matter what the day looks like—raining, foggy, overcast, sunny—my heart swells with gratitude. I get another chance.
> - Oprah Winfrey

AN ATTITUDE OF GRATITUDE KEEPS YOU GOING WHEN THINGS ARE TOUGH.

I AM GRATEFUL FOR...

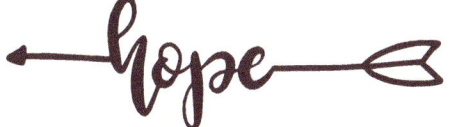

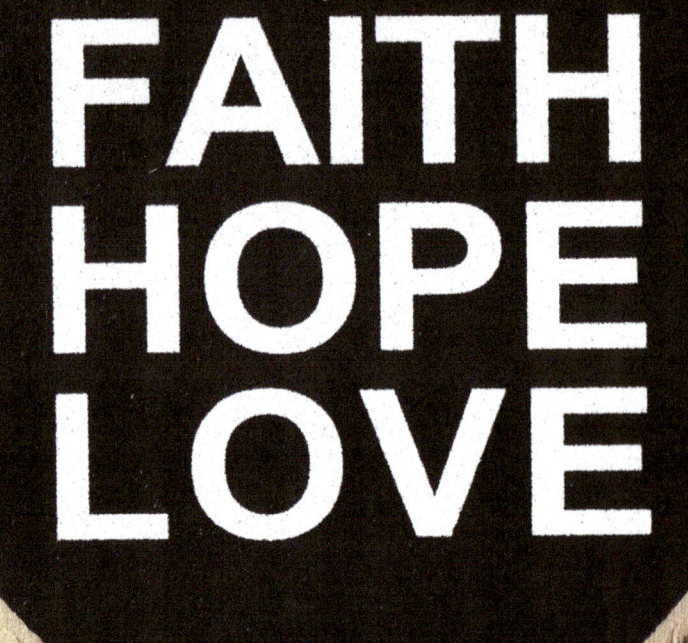

AN ATTITUDE OF GRATITUDE IMPROVES YOUR SLEEP.

I AM GRATEFUL FOR...

hope

*"When I let go of what I am,
I become what I might be."*
—Lao Tzu

AN ATTITUDE OF GRATITUDE HELPS YOU STAY IN THE PRESENT MOMENT.

I AM GRATEFUL FOR...

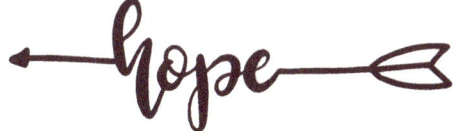

Start everyday with attitude of gratitude.

THE MORE YOU FOCUS ON YOUR BLESSINGS, THE MORE BLESSINGS YOU SHALL RECEIVE.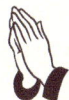

I AM GRATEFUL FOR...

hope

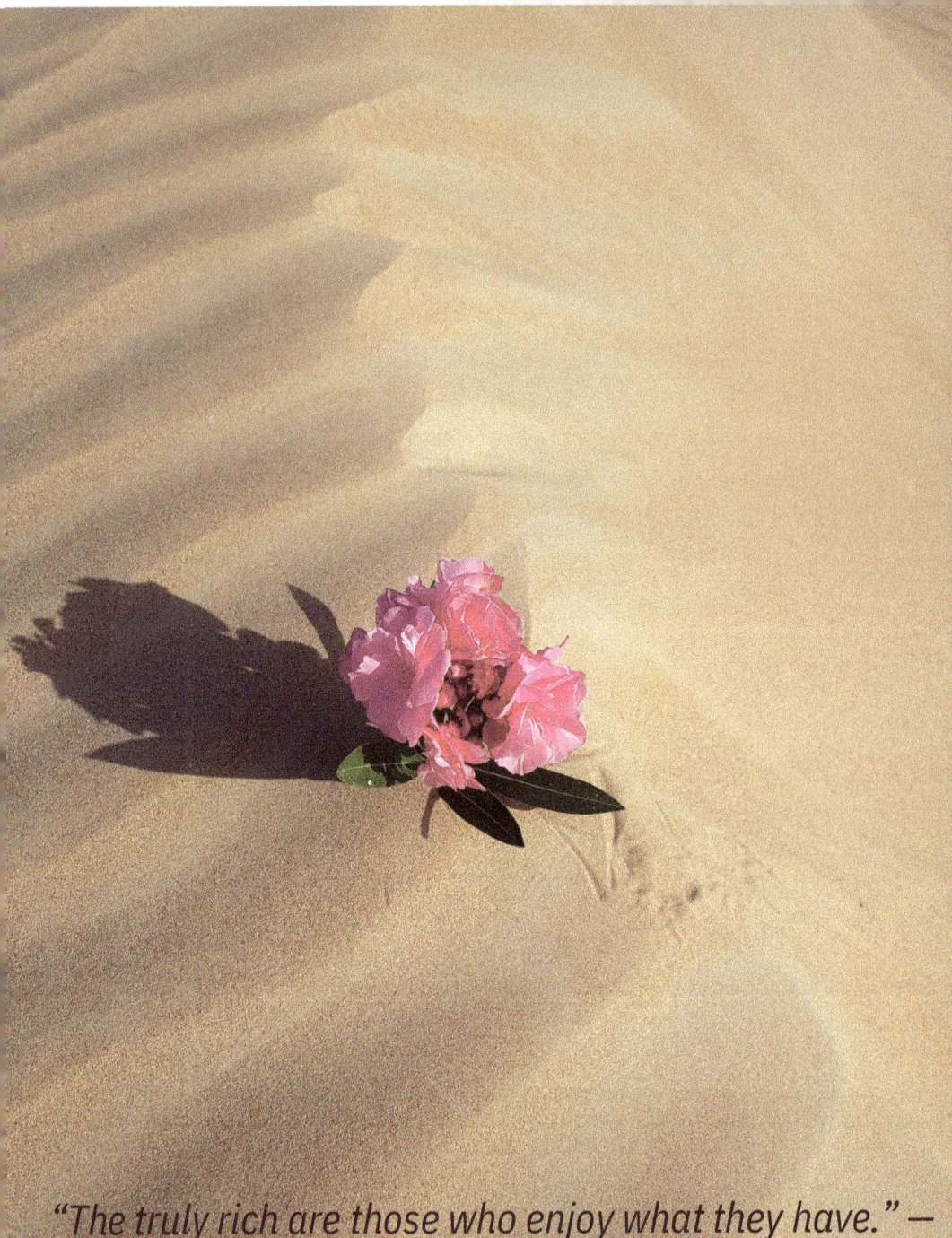

"The truly rich are those who enjoy what they have." — Yiddish Proverb

THROUGH THE EYES OF GRATITUDE, EVERYTHING IS A MIRACLE.

I AM GRATEFUL FOR...

hope

"Do not allow people to dim your shine because they are blinded. Tell them to put some sunglasses on."

IF YOU WANT TO BE HAPPY, LEARN TO BE GRATEFUL.

I AM GRATEFUL FOR...

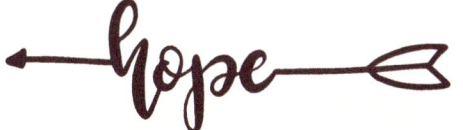

"In case no one has told you, you are amazing, strong, brave, loved, worthy, and unique.
There is no one like you.
The world needs you."

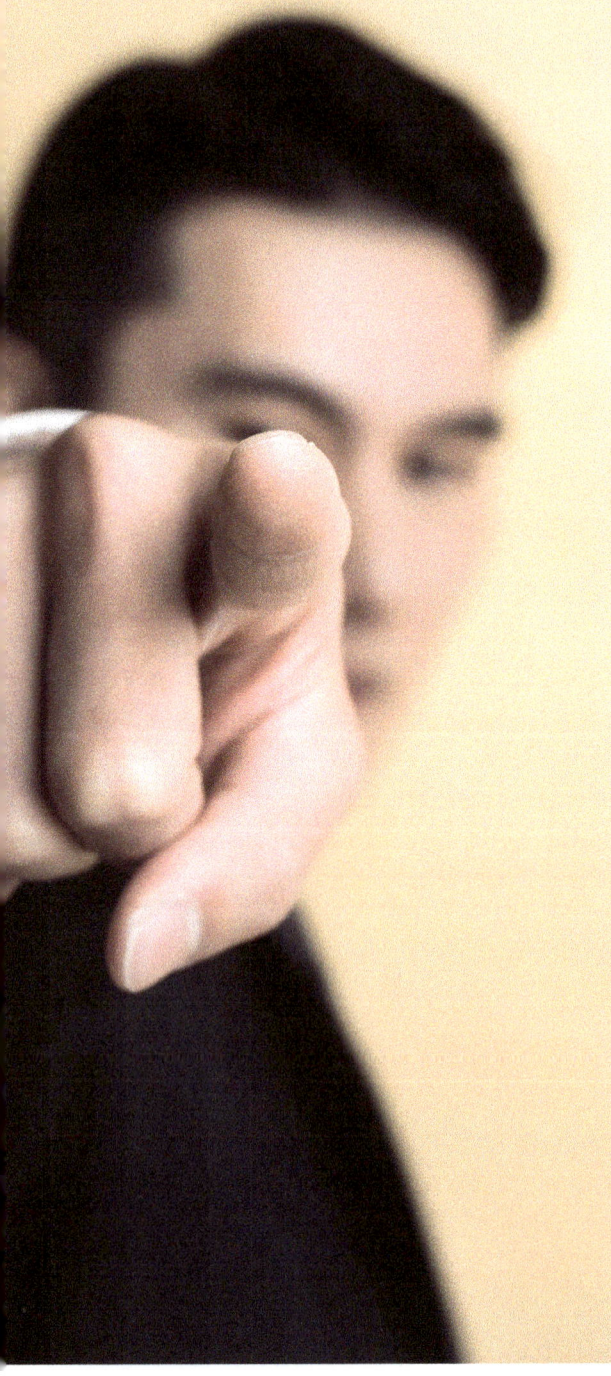

THANKSGIVING DOES NOT HAVE TO BE JUST ONE DAY. IT SHOULD BE EVERY DAY.

I AM GRATEFUL FOR...

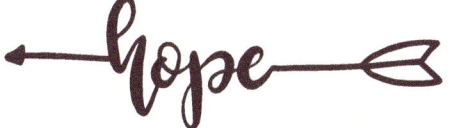

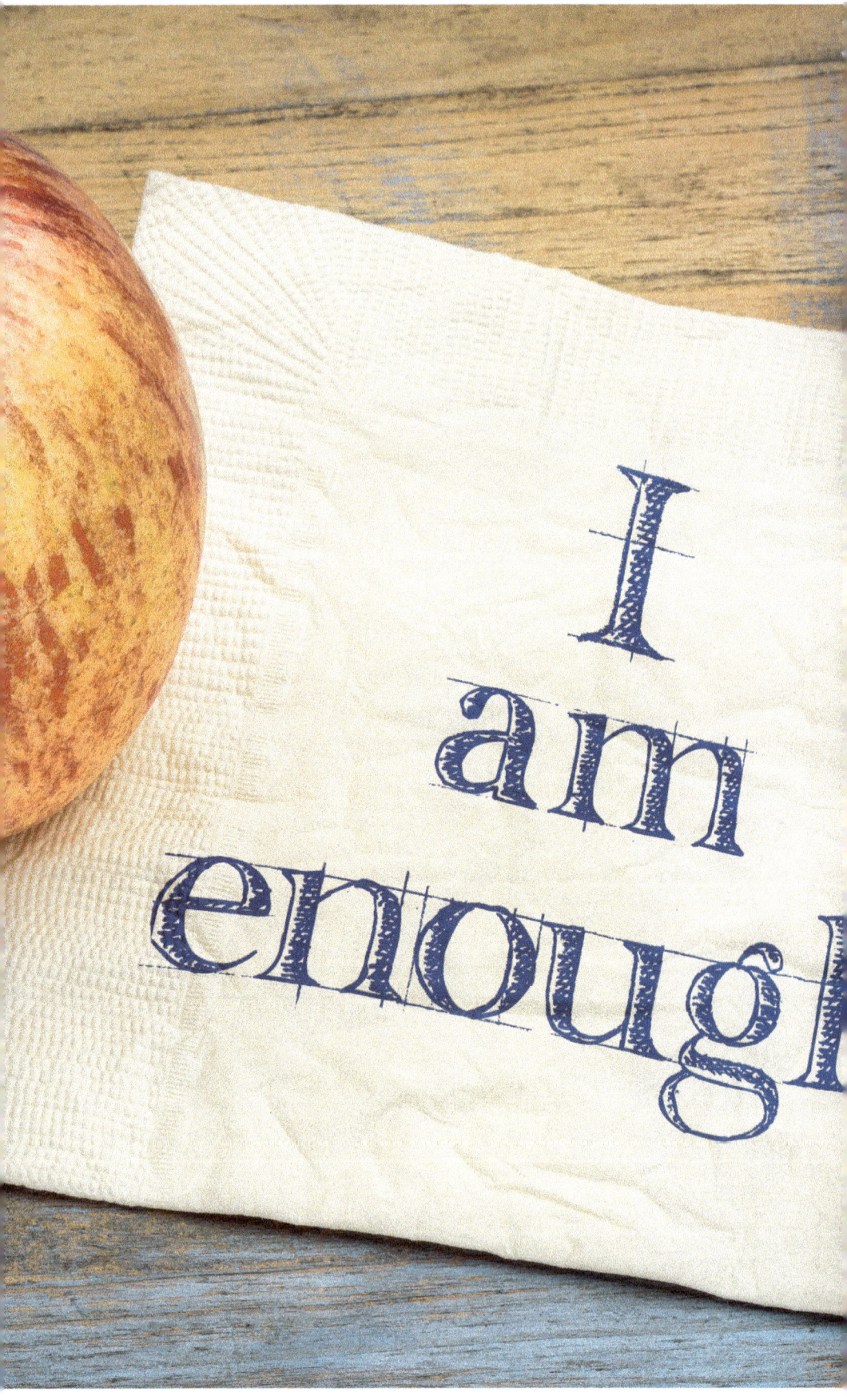

"WHEN EATING FRUIT, REMEMBER THE ONE WHO PLANTED THE TREE."

I AM GRATEFUL FOR...

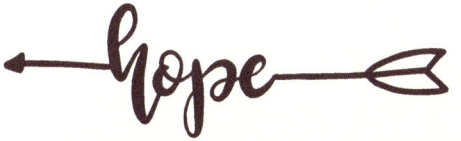

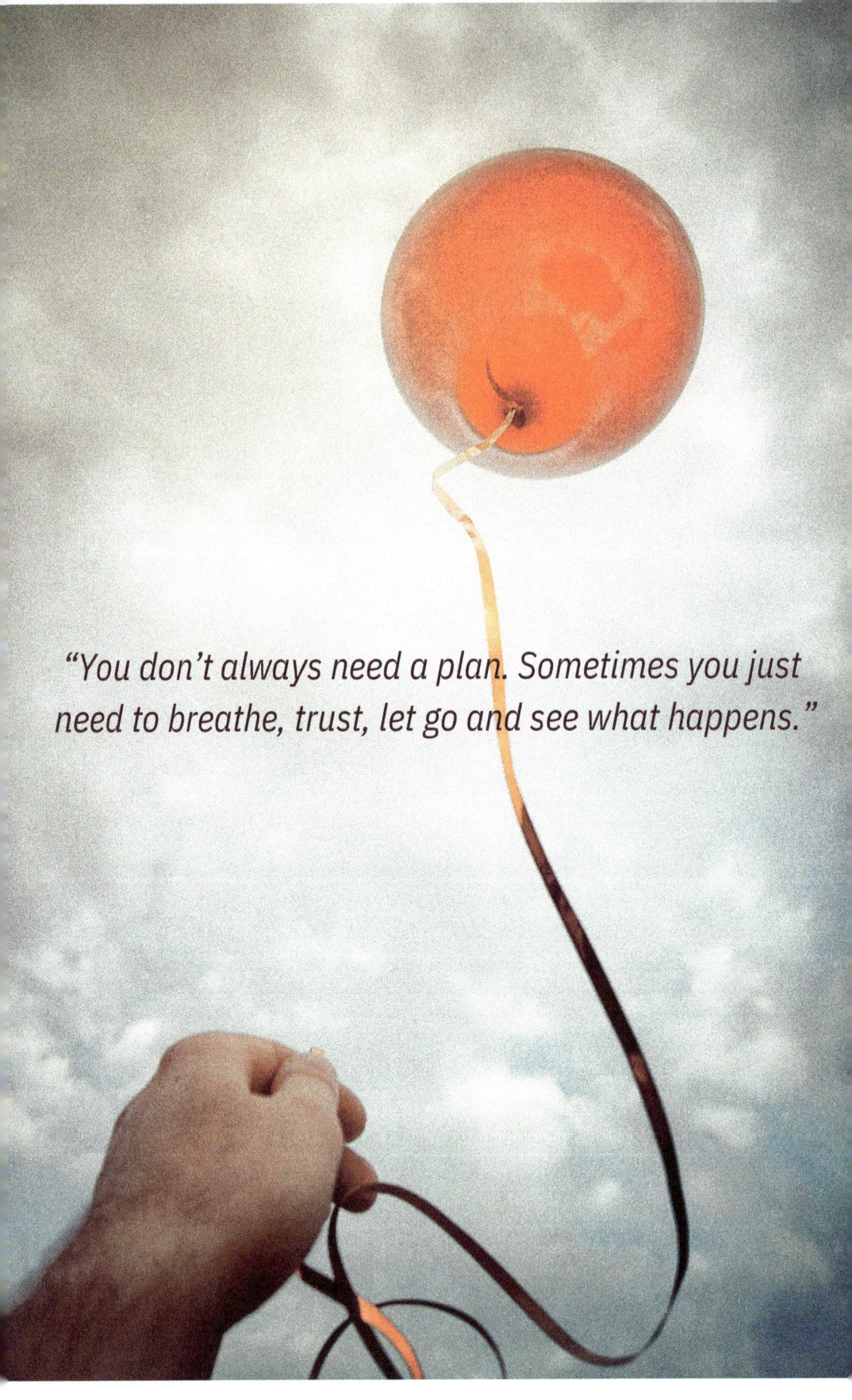

"WHEN EATING FRUIT, REMEMBER THE ONE WHO PLANTED THE TREE."

I AM GRATEFUL FOR...

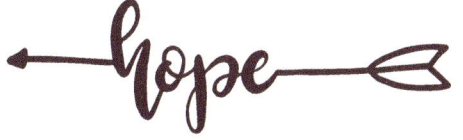

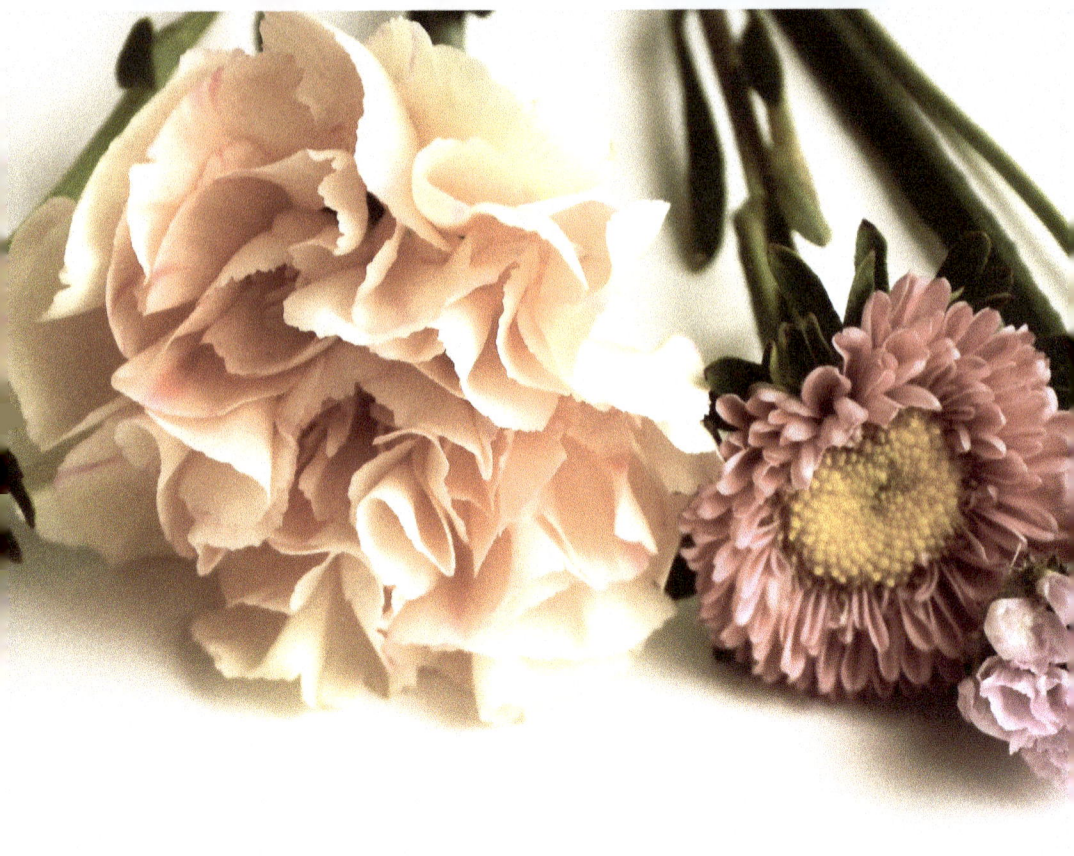

Dream

When the dream is big enough facts don't count.

"WEAR GRATITUDE LIKE A CLOAK, AND IT WILL FEED EVERY CORNER OF YOUR LIFE." RUMI."

I AM GRATEFUL FOR...

"Nature does not hurry yet everything is accomplished."
- Lao Tzu

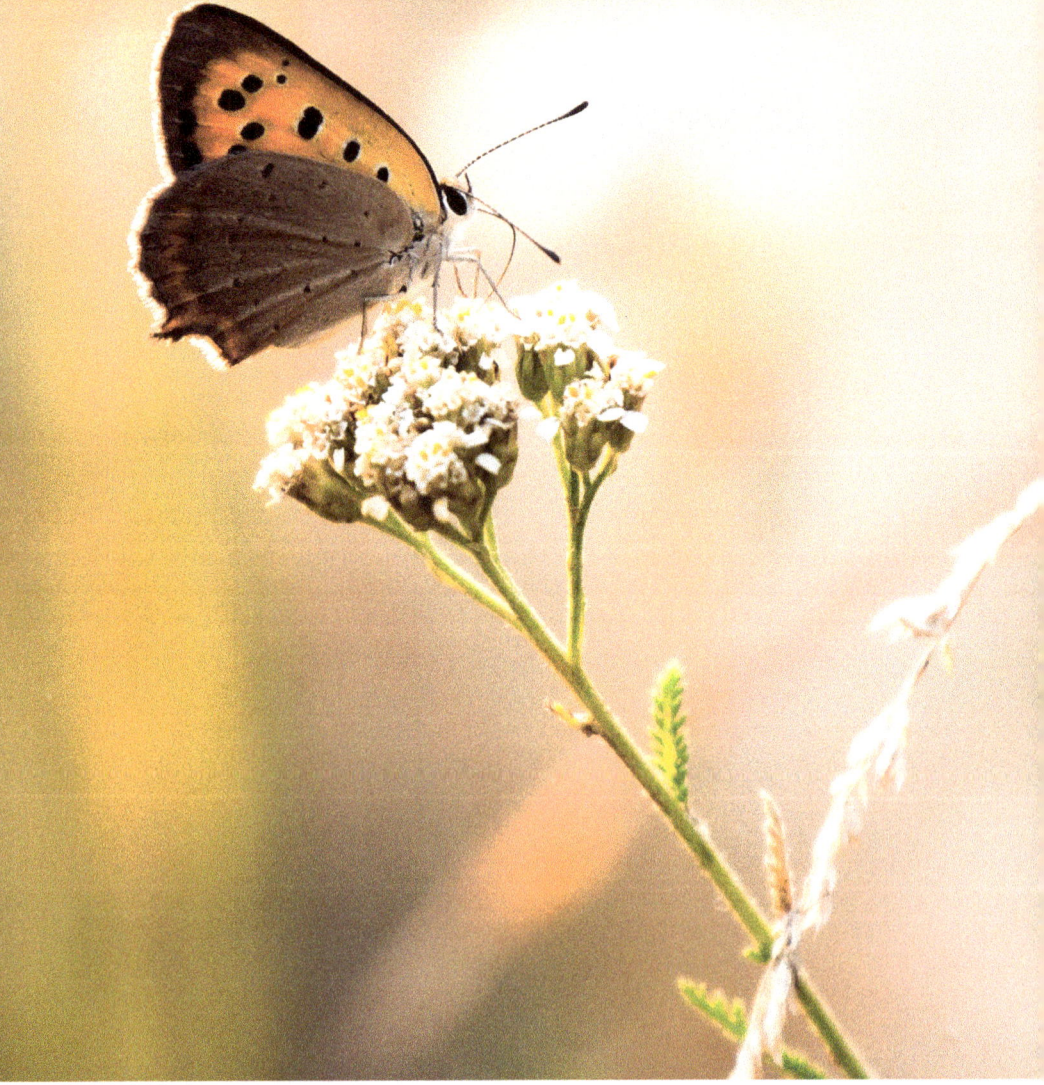

WHEN YOU CHANGE THE WAY YOU LOOK AT THINGS, THINGS YOU LOOK AT CHANGE. COUNT YOUR BLESSINGS EVEN IN TOUGH TIMES.

I AM GRATEFUL FOR...

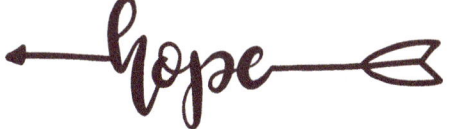

"Knowing others is intelligence; knowing yourself is true wisdom. Mastering others is strength; mastering yourself is true power." - Lao Tsu

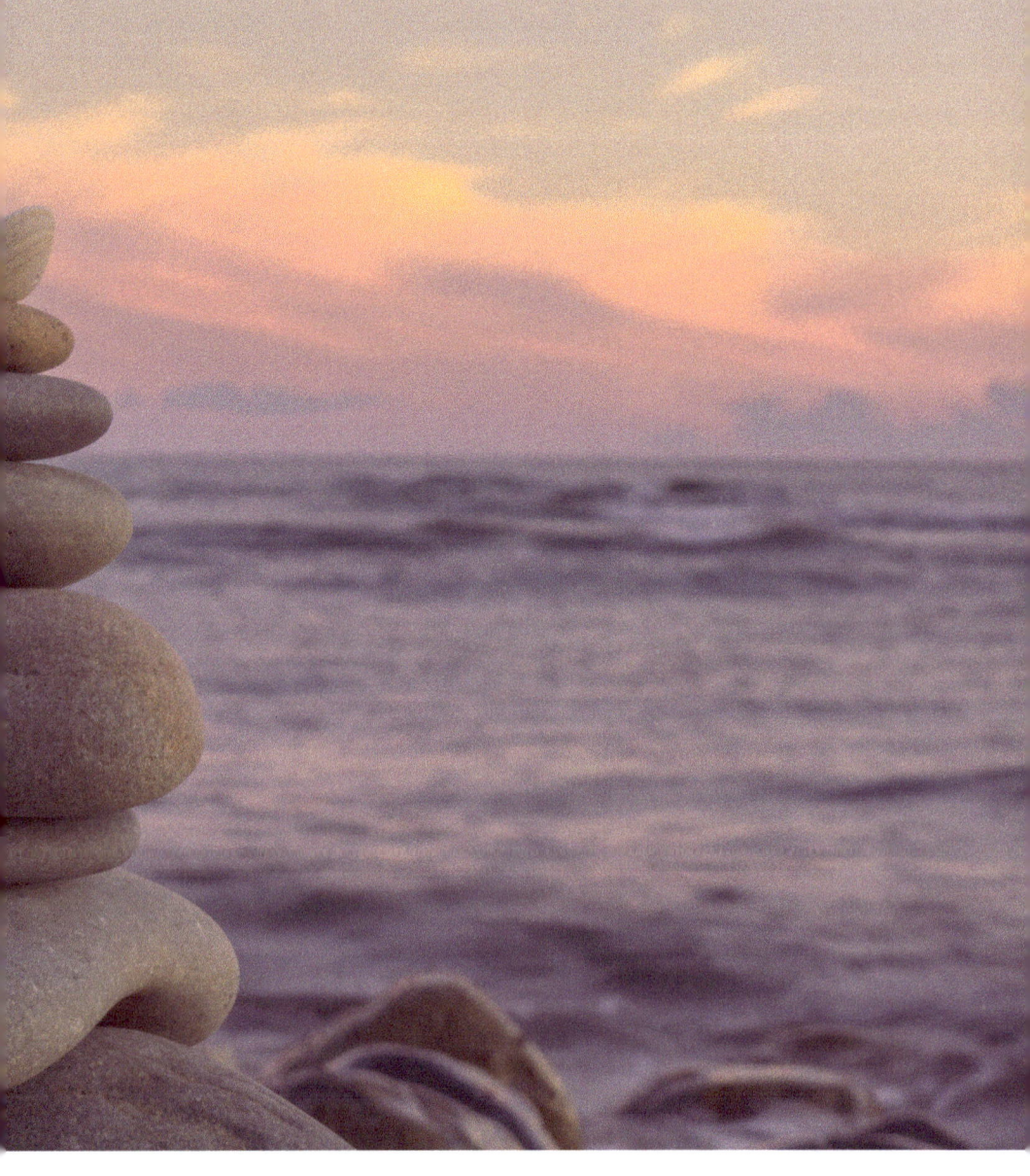

AN ATTITUDE OF GRATITUDE INCREASES YOUR FAITH IN THE UNIVERSE AND CALMS YOUR MIND.

I AM GRATEFUL FOR...

hope

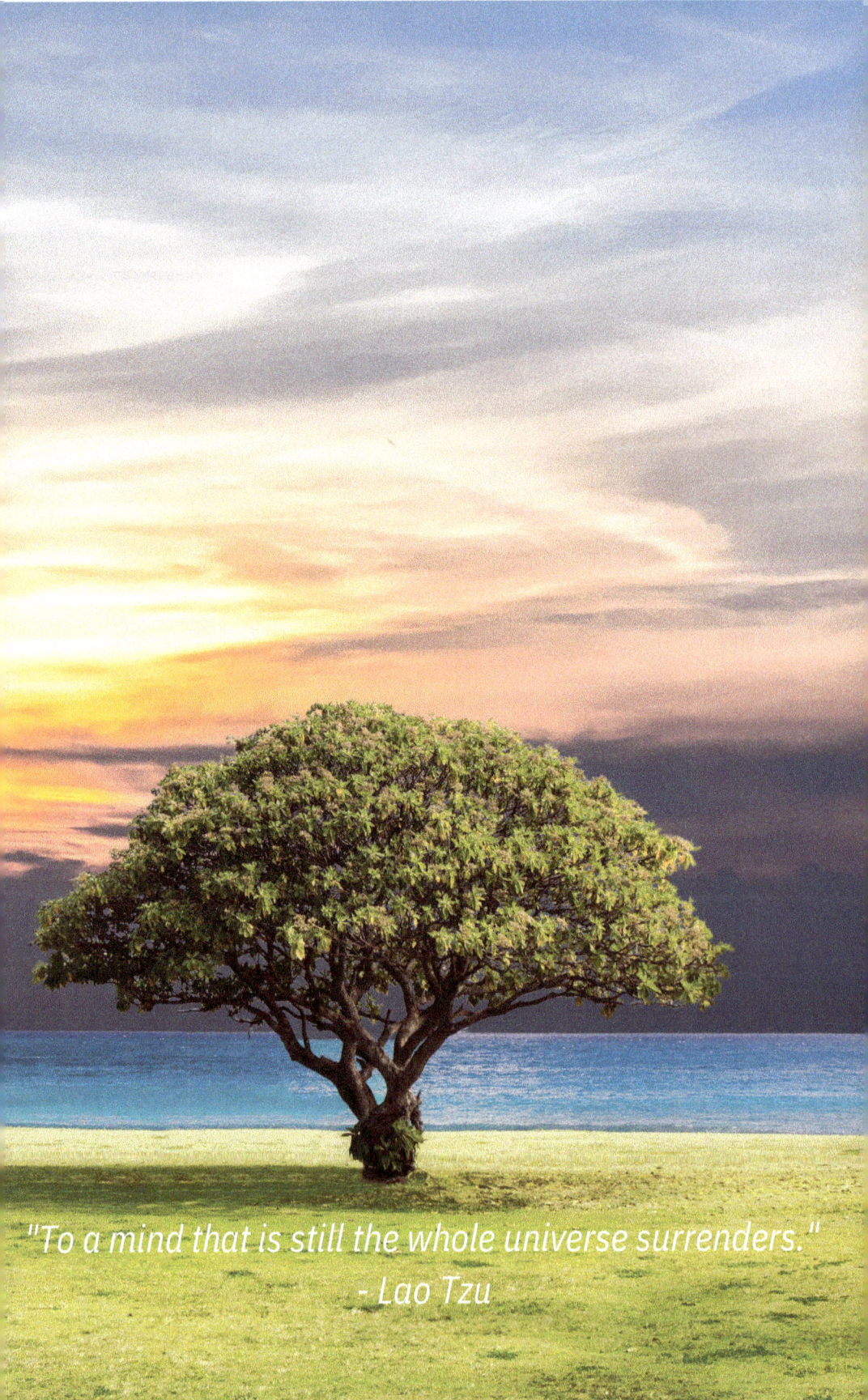

GRATITUDE AND ATTITUDE ARE NOT CHALLENGES. THEY ARE CHOICES.

I AM GRATEFUL FOR...

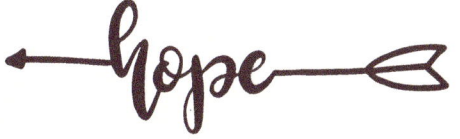

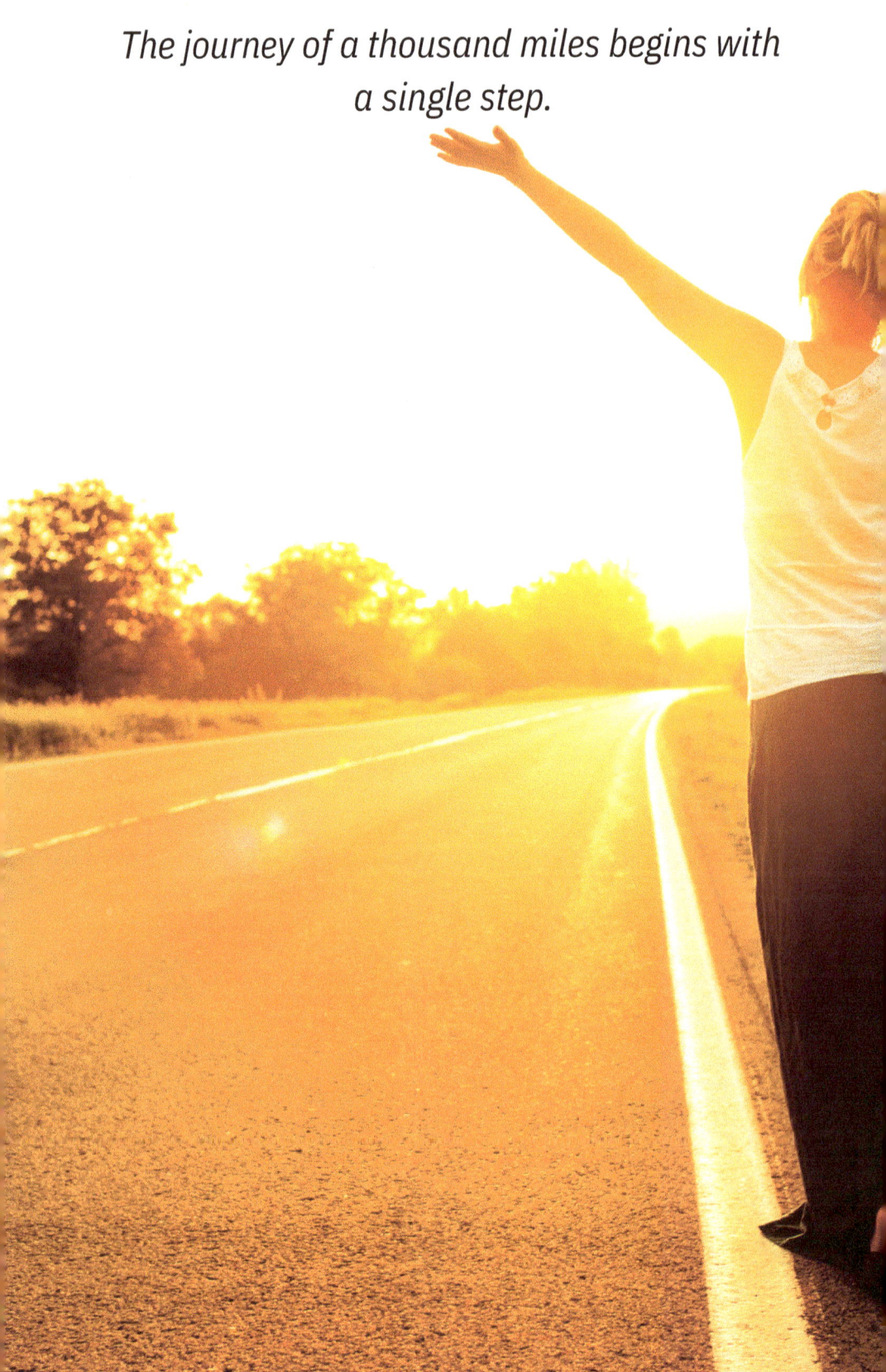

The journey of a thousand miles begins with a single step.

" IF A FELLOW ISN'T THANKFUL FOR WHAT HE'S GOT, HE ISN'T LIKELY TO BE THANKFUL FOR WHAT HE'S GOING TO GET." — FRANK A. CLARK

I AM GRATEFUL FOR...

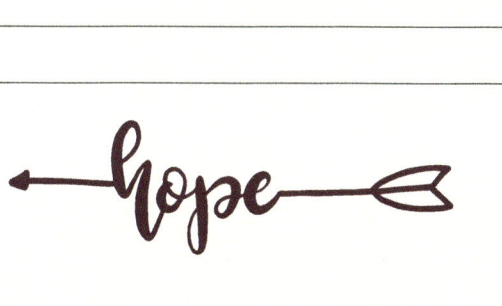

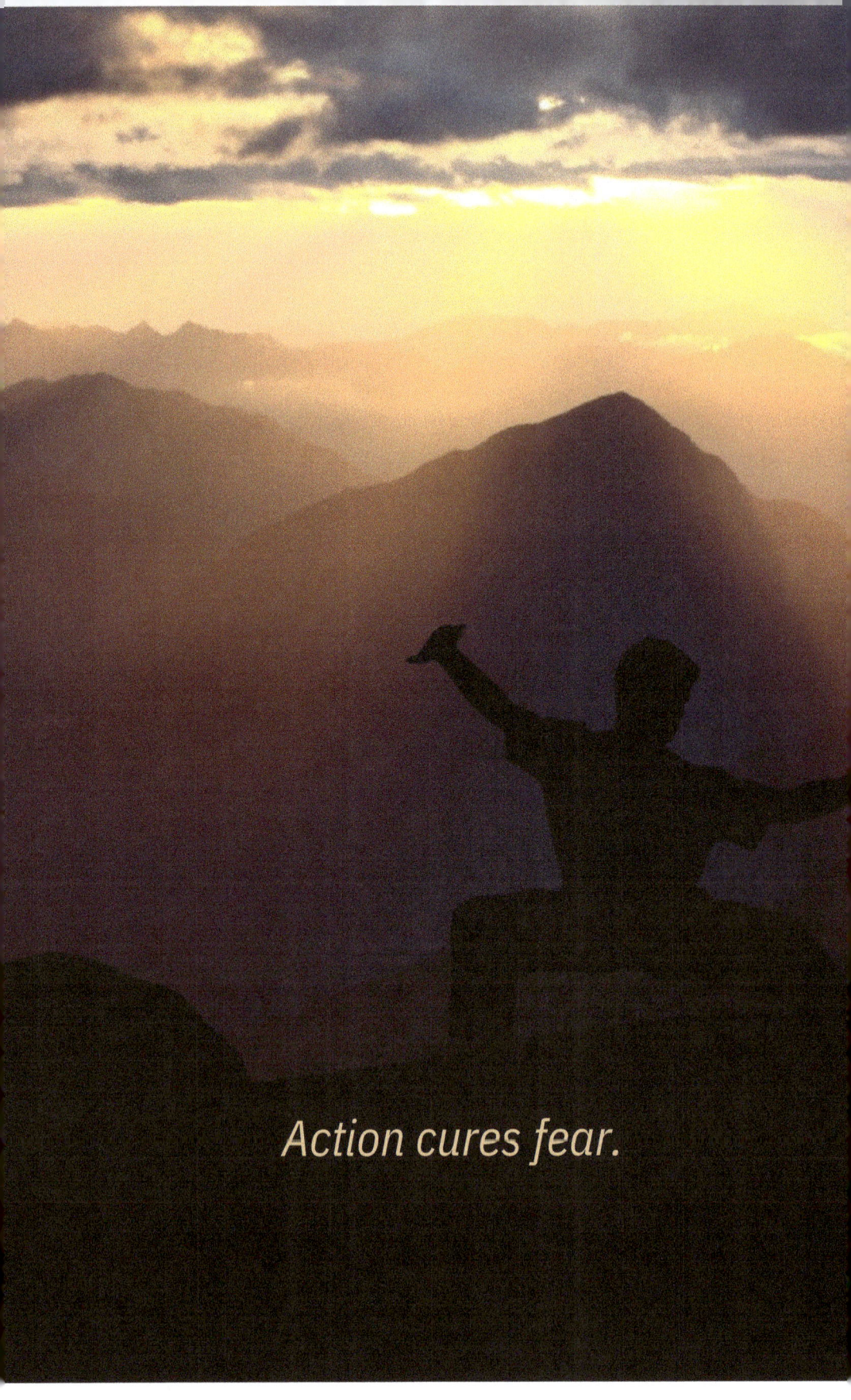

EXPRESS GRATITUDE NOT ONLY BY YOUR WORDS BUT THROUGH YOUR ACTIONS AS WELL.

I AM GRATEFUL FOR...

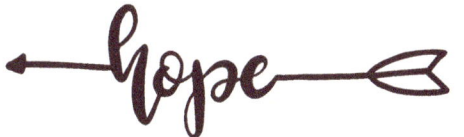

*Watch your thoughts, they become your words;
watch your words, they become your actions;
watch your actions, they become your habits;
watch your habits, they become your character;
watch your character, it becomes your destiny.*

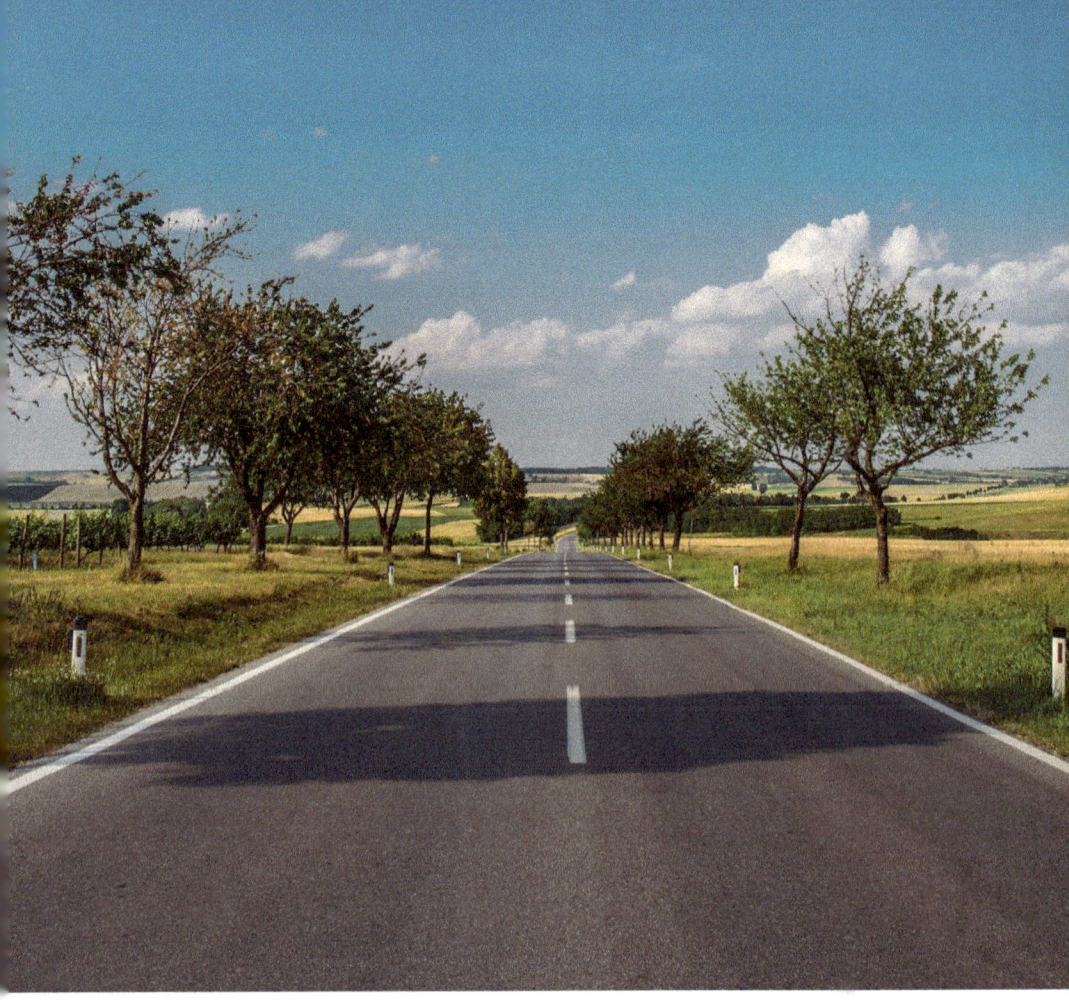

NOT ONLY COUNT YOUR BLESSINGS BUT BE A BLESSING IN SOMEONE'S LIFE.

I AM GRATEFUL FOR...

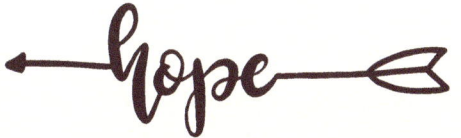

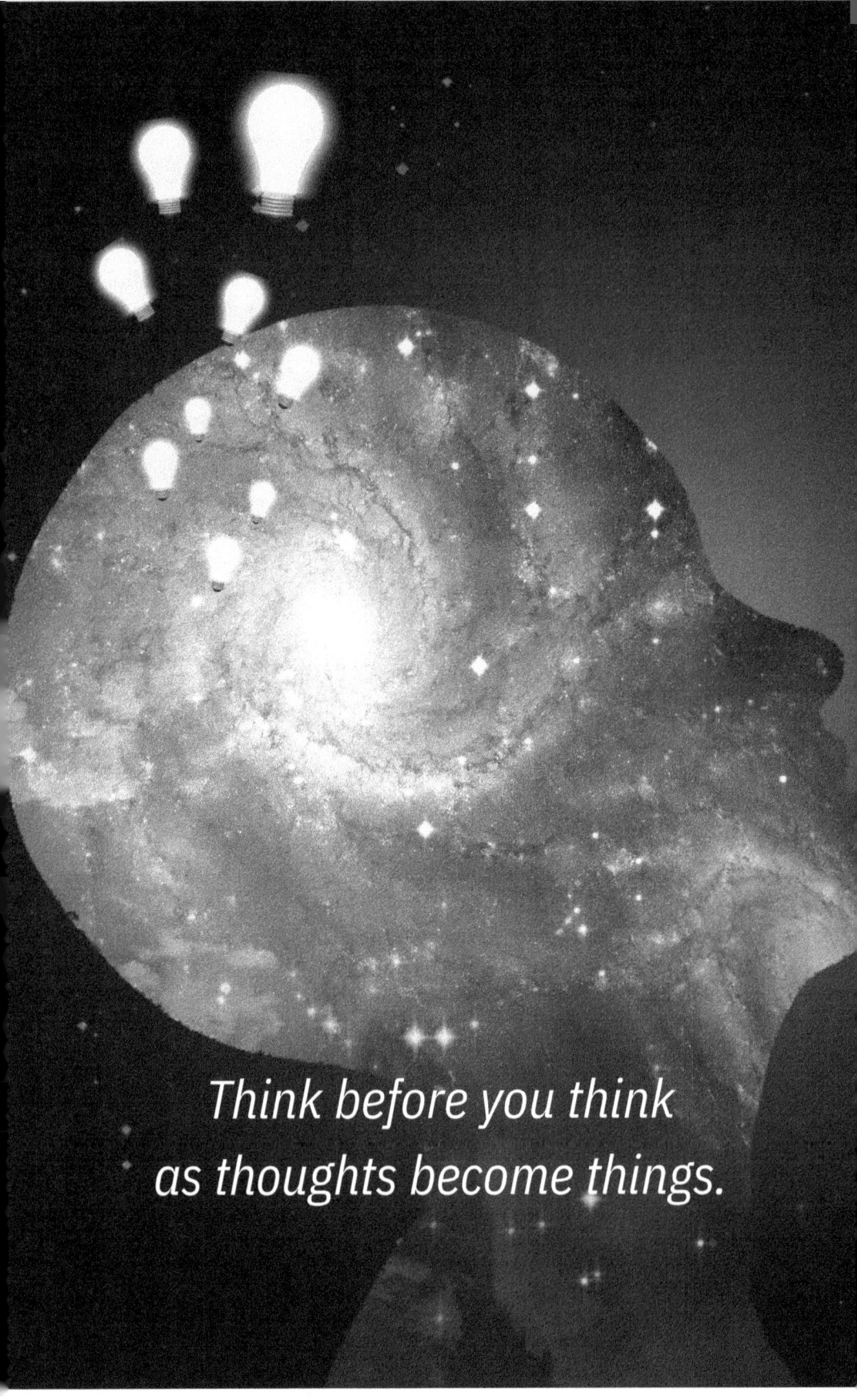

WHEN YOU ARE HAPPY WITH WHAT YOU HAVE, YOU WILL RECEIVE MORE THINGS TO BE HAPPY ABOUT.

I AM GRATEFUL FOR...

hope

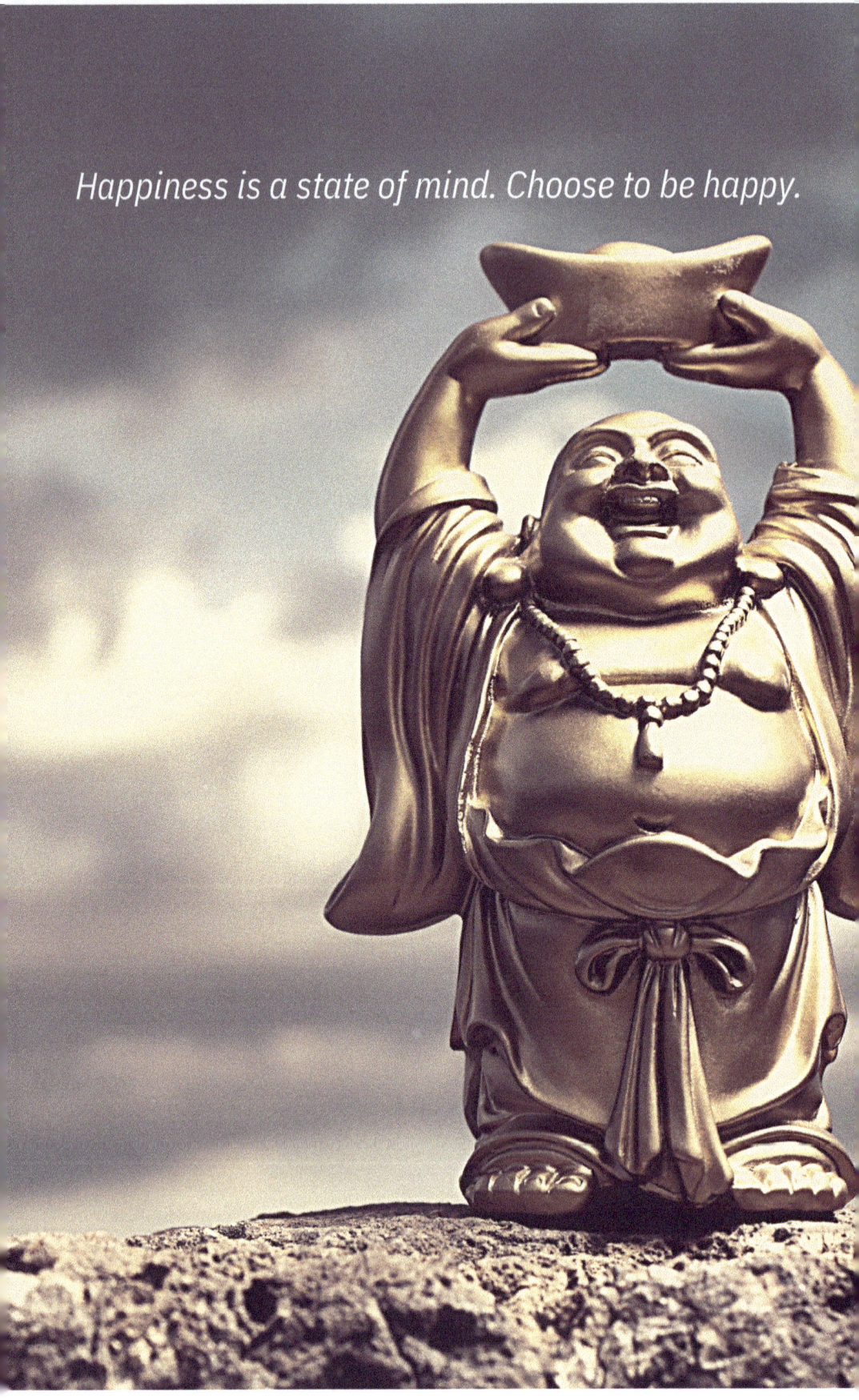

AN ATTITUDE OF GRATITUDE IS THE ENEMY OF DISCONTENT AND DISSATISFACTION.

I AM GRATEFUL FOR...

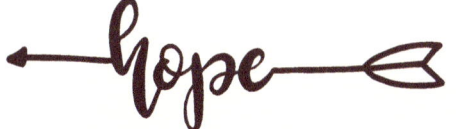

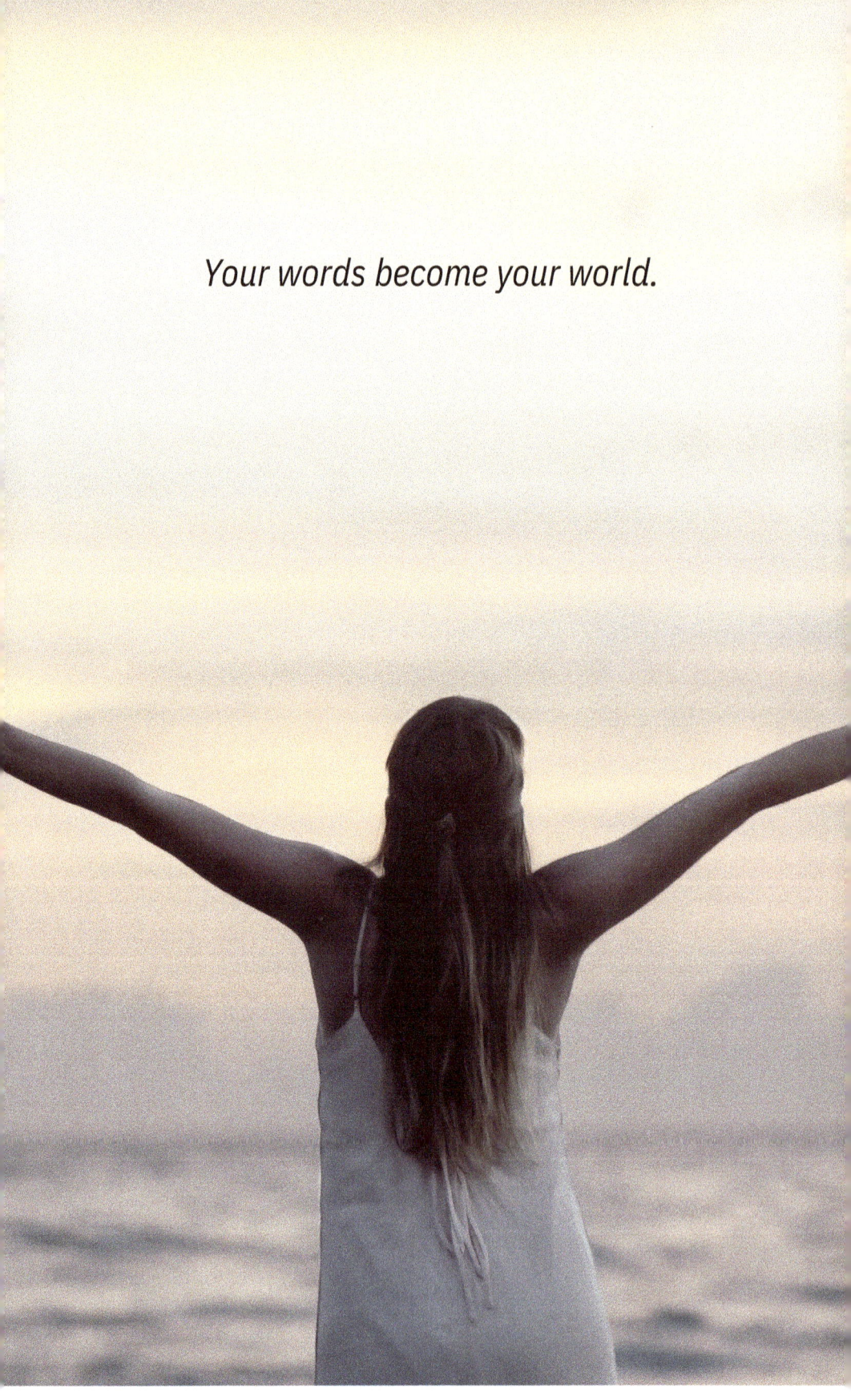

"FEELING GRATITUDE AND NOT EXPRESSING IT IS LIKE WRAPPING A PRESENT AND NOT GIVING IT." WILLIAM ARTHUR WARD

I AM GRATEFUL FOR...

hope

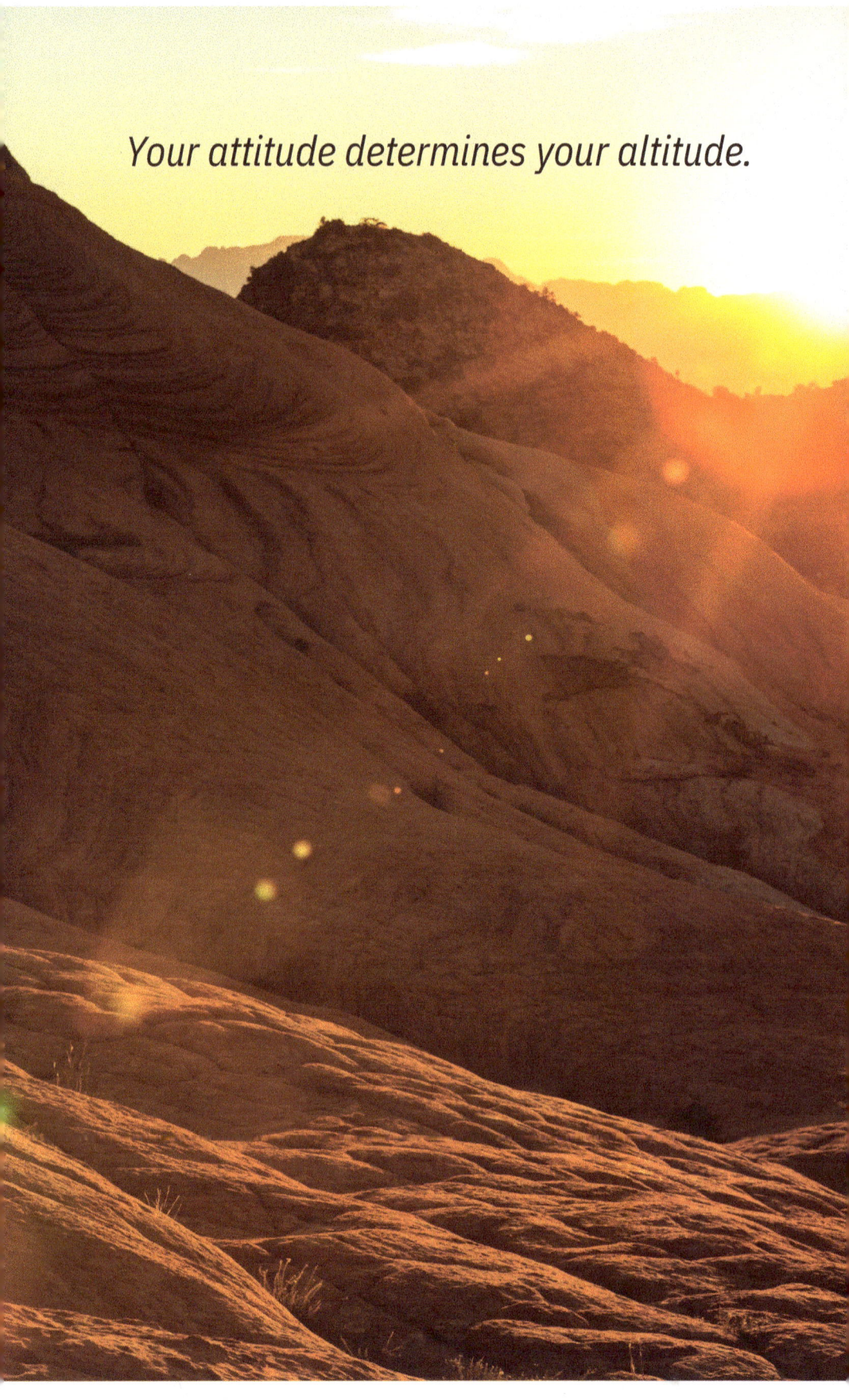

"IF YOU COUNT ALL YOUR ASSETS, YOU ALWAYS SHOW A PROFIT." ROBERT QUILLEN

I AM GRATEFUL FOR...

hope

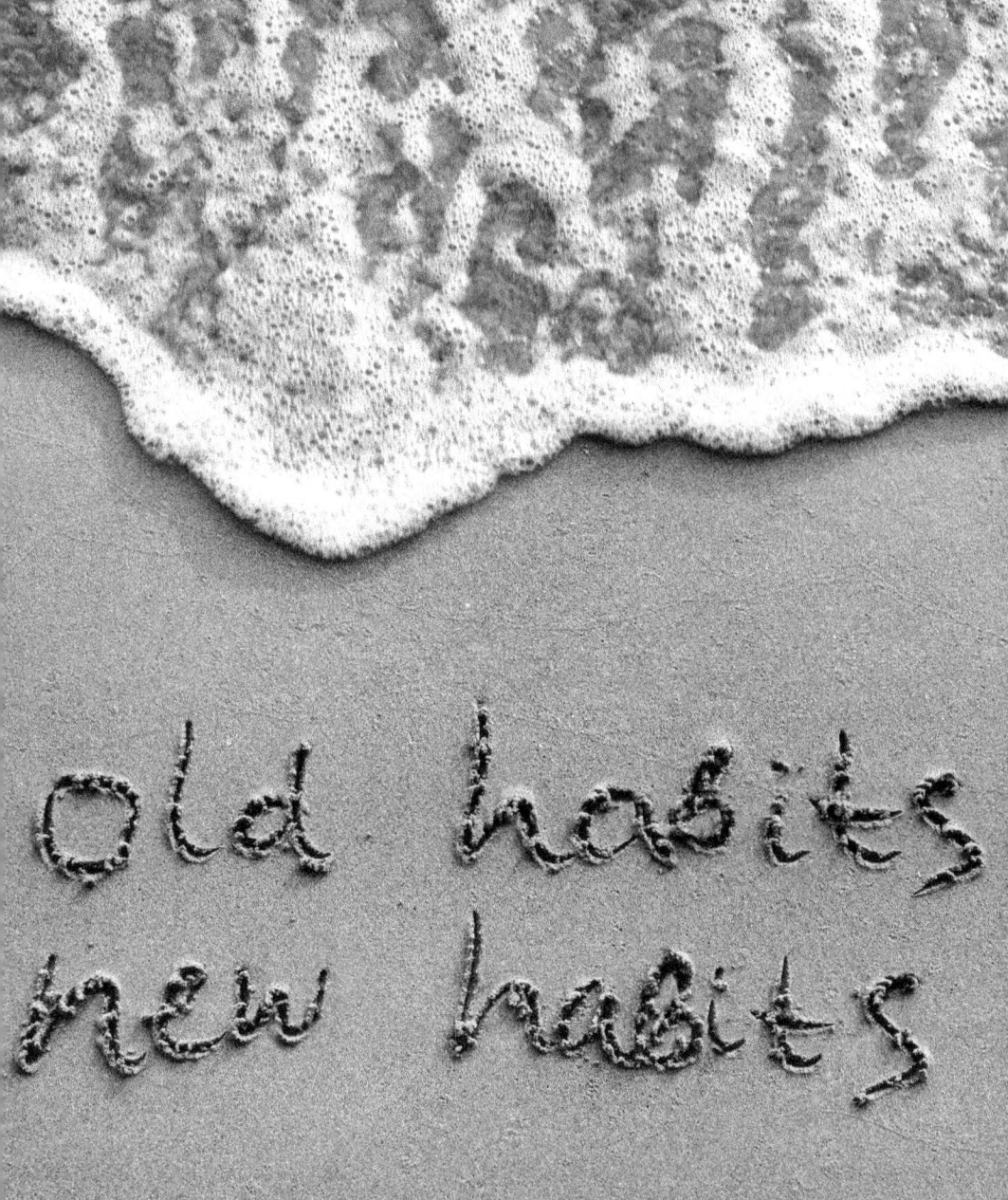

"ACKNOWLEDGING THE GOOD THAT YOU ALREADY HAVE IN YOUR LIFE IS THE FOUNDATION FOR ALL ABUNDANCE."
ECKHART TOLLE

I AM GRATEFUL FOR...

hope

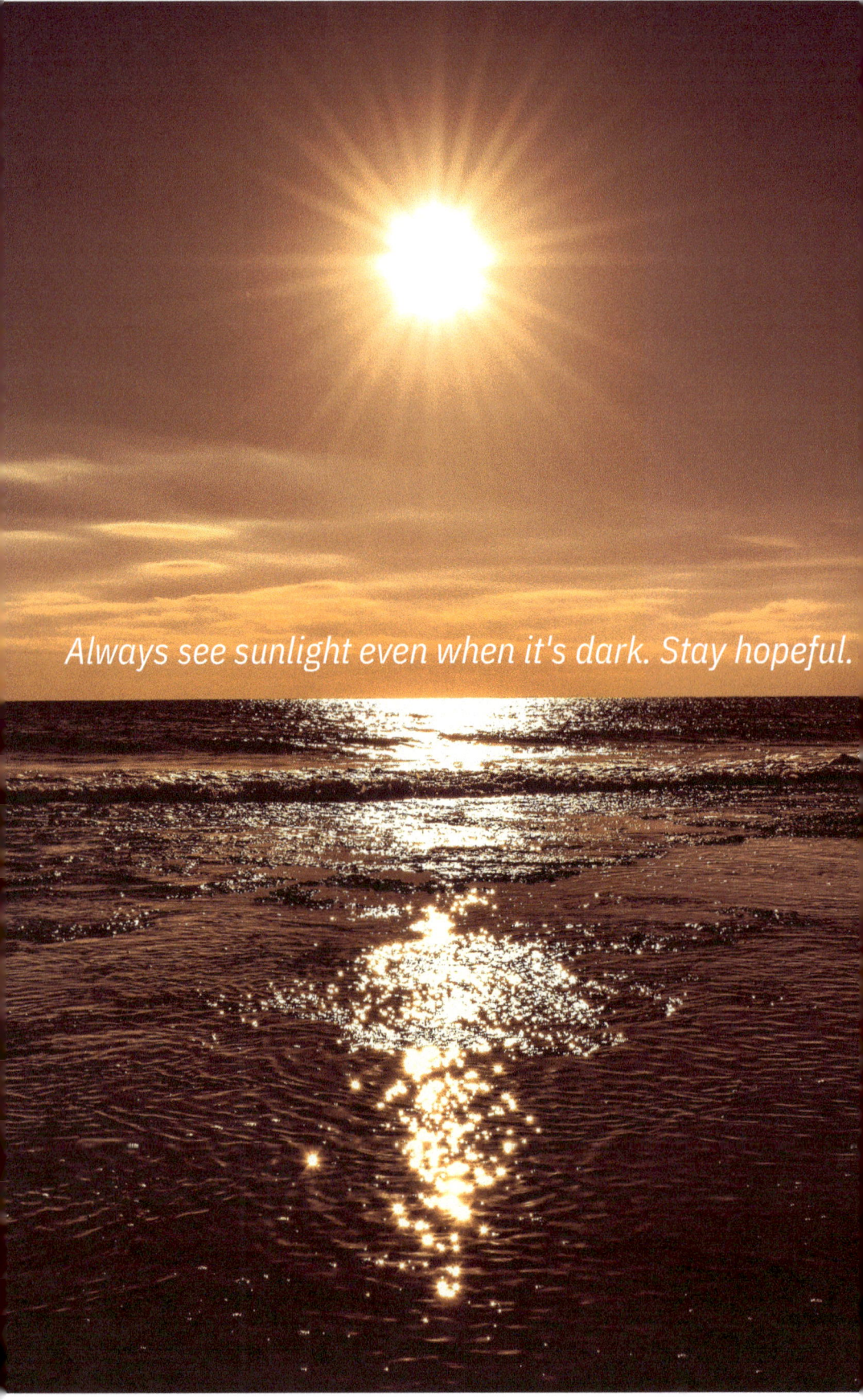

"GRATITUDE IS A CURRENCY THAT WE CAN MINT FOR OURSELVES, AND SPEND WITHOUT FEAR OF BANKRUPTCY."
FRED DE WITT VAN AMBURGH

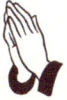

I AM GRATEFUL FOR...

hope

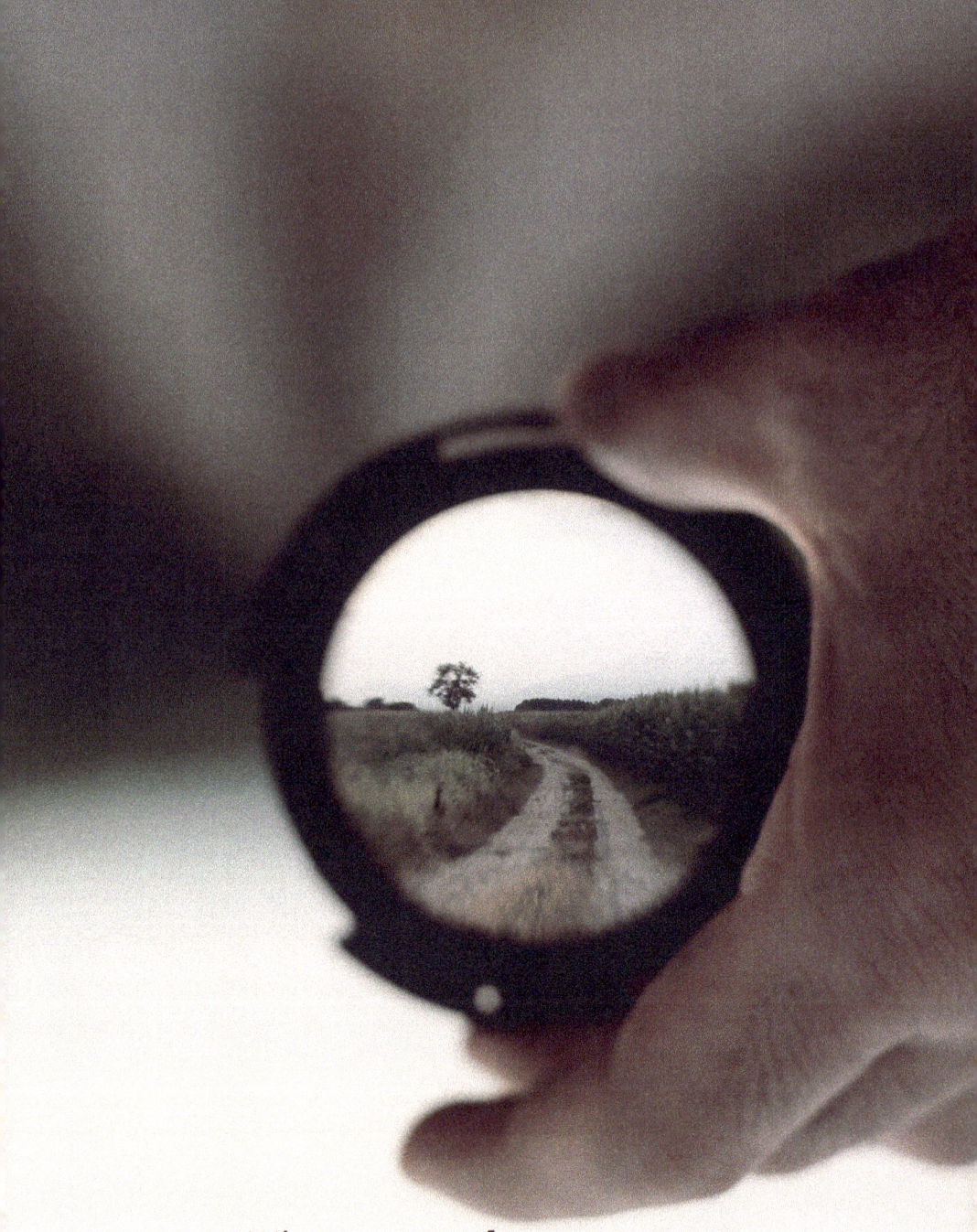

Whatever you focus on, grows.
If you focus on your problems, your problems will grow.
If you focus on the solutions, your problems will shrink.

"IT IS IMPOSSIBLE TO FEEL GRATEFUL AND UNHAPPY IN THE SAME MOMENT."

I AM GRATEFUL FOR...

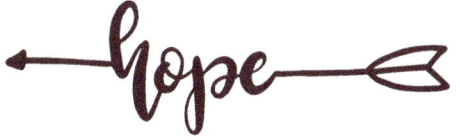

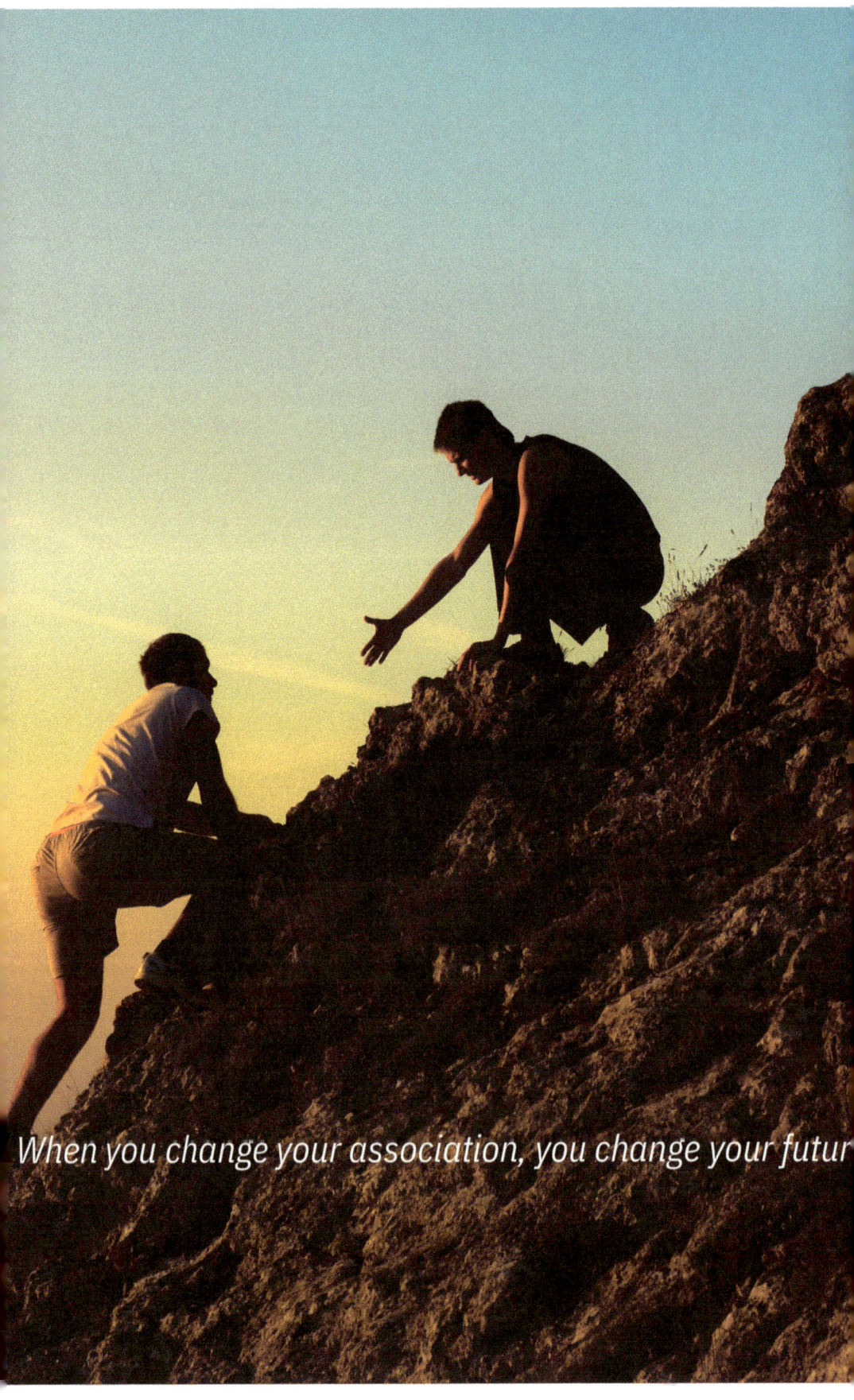

"THINGS TURN OUT BEST FOR PEOPLE WHO MAKE THE BEST OF THE WAY THINGS TURN OUT." JOHN WOODEN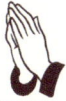

I AM GRATEFUL FOR...

hope

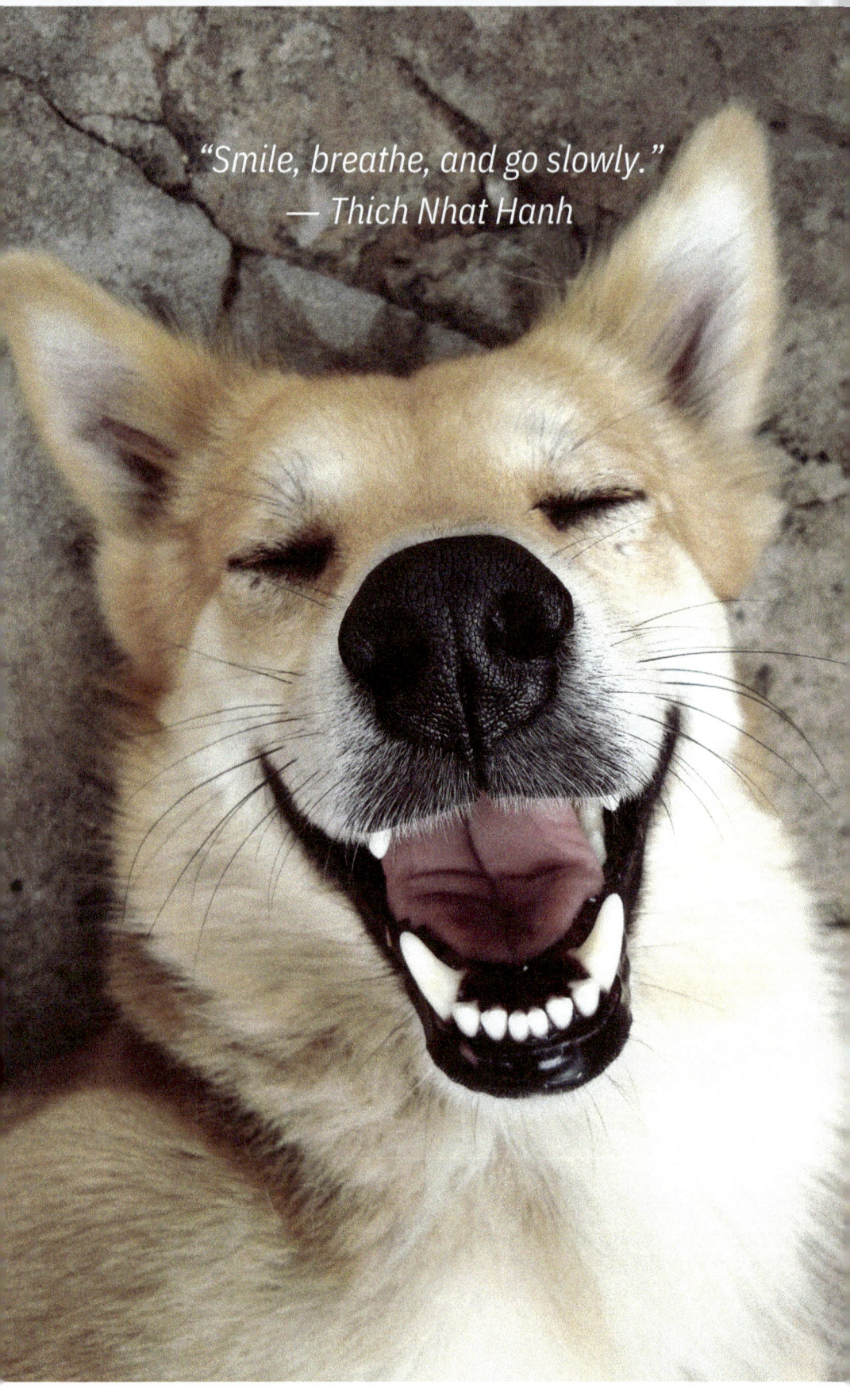

"FORGET YESTERDAY. IT HAS ALREADY FORGOTTEN YOU. DON'T SWEAT TOMORROW. YOU HAVEN'T EVEN MET. INSTEAD, OPEN YOUR EYES AND YOUR HEART TO A TRULY PRECIOUS GIFT— TODAY." STEVE MARABOLI

I AM GRATEFUL FOR...

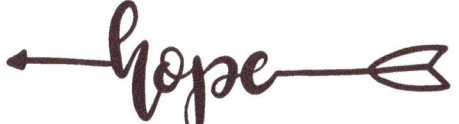

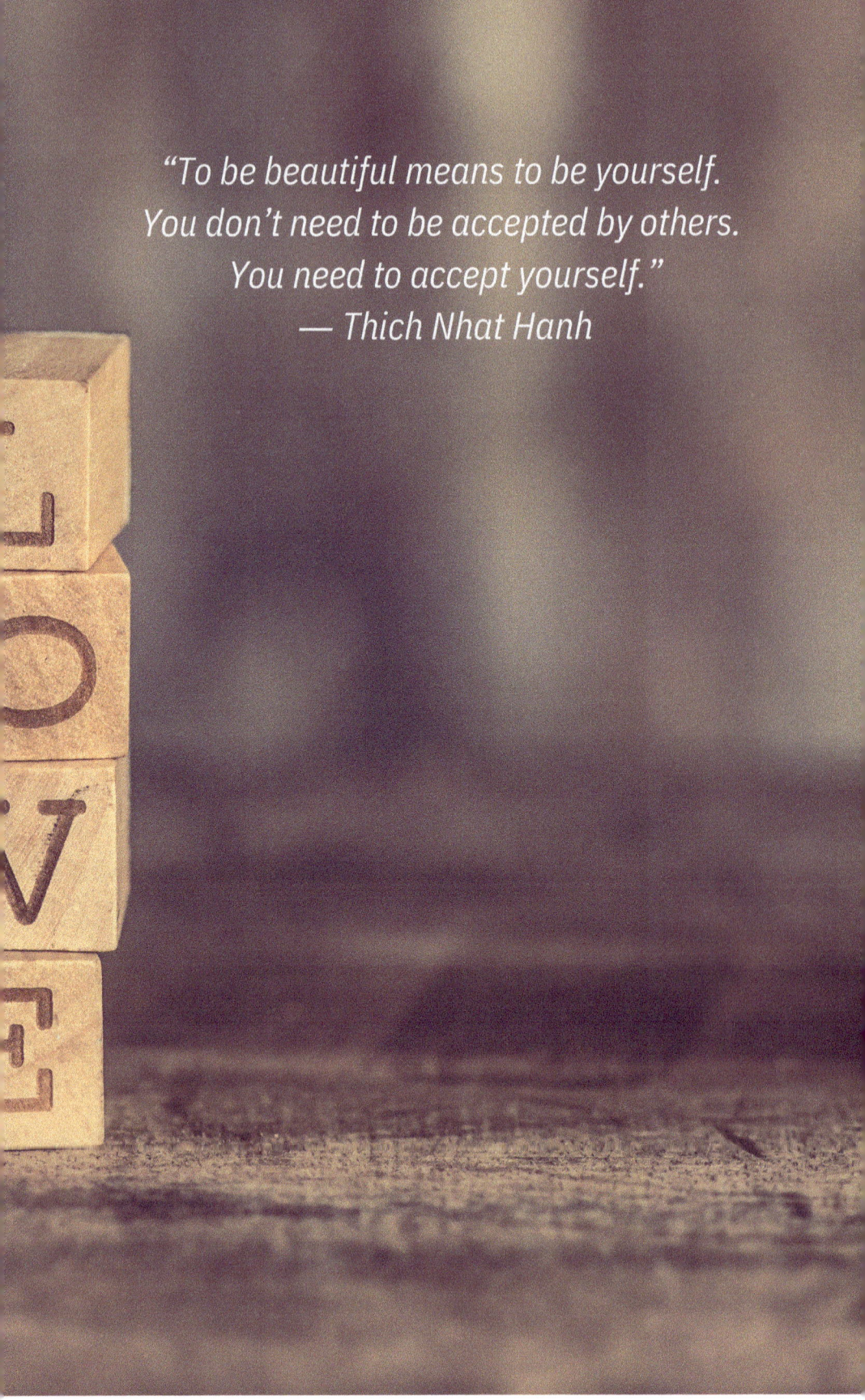

"To be beautiful means to be yourself.
You don't need to be accepted by others.
You need to accept yourself."
— Thich Nhat Hanh

"GRATITUDE ALSO OPENS YOUR EYES TO THE LIMITLESS POTENTIAL OF THE UNIVERSE, WHILE DISSATISFACTION CLOSES YOUR EYES TO IT." STEPHEN RICHARDS

I AM GRATEFUL FOR...

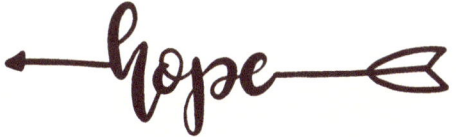

"Sometimes your joy is the source of your smile, but sometimes your smile can be the source of your joy."
— Thich Nhat Hanh

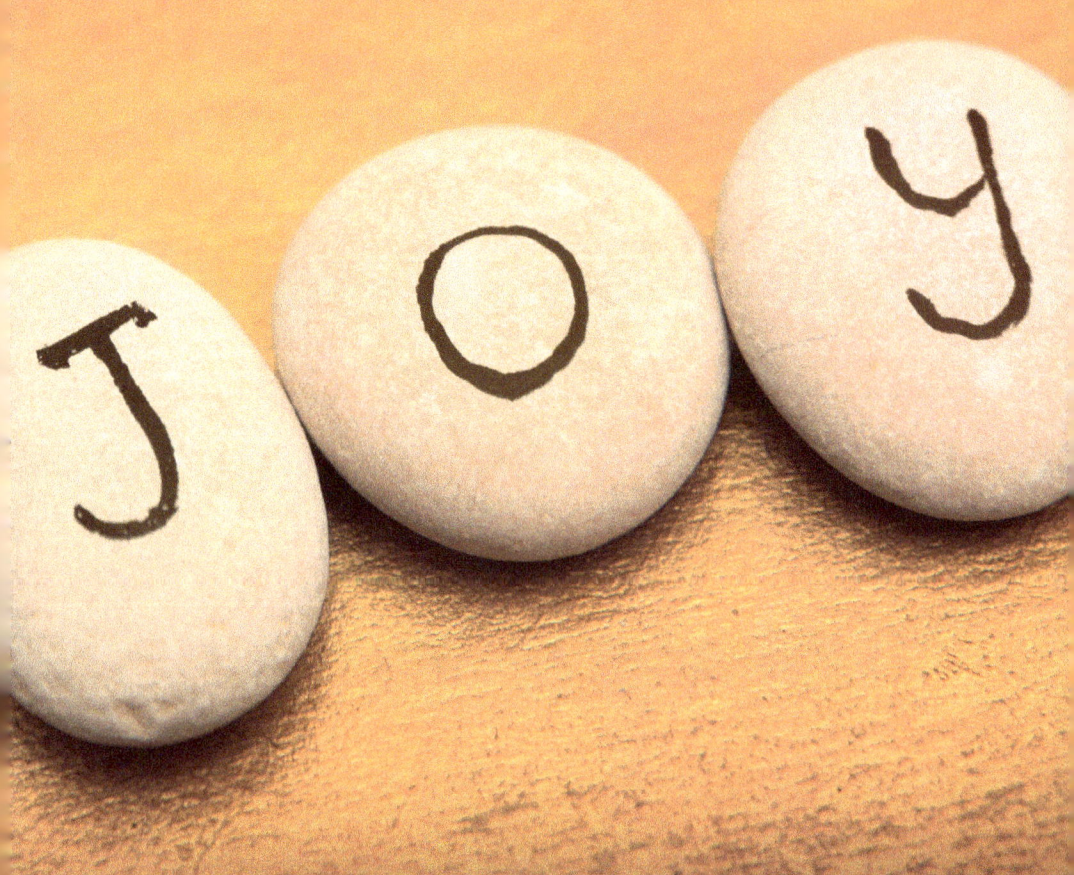

"COUNT YOUR BLESSINGS AND MAKE YOUR BLESSINGS COUNT."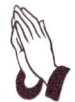

I AM GRATEFUL FOR...

hope

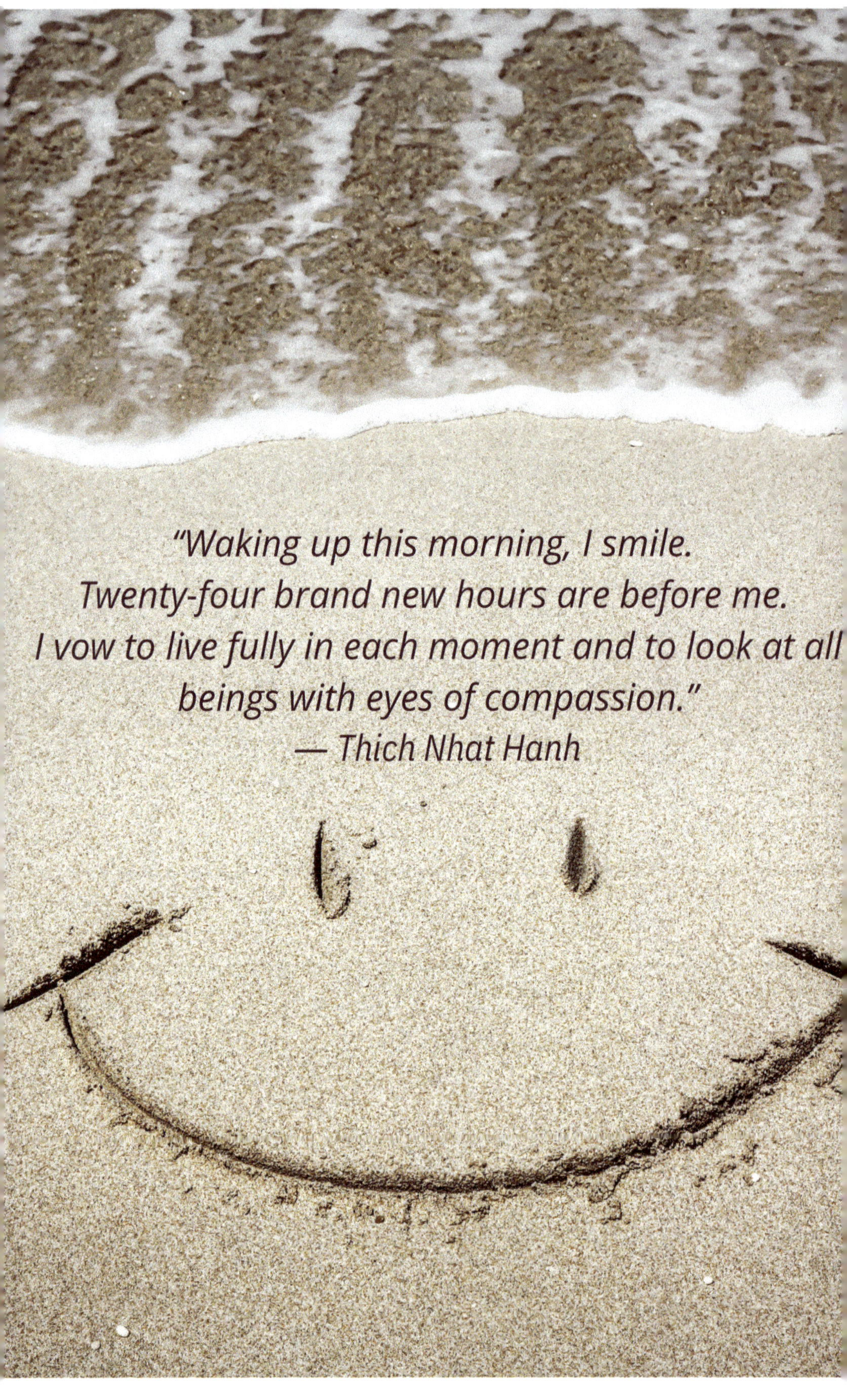

"Waking up this morning, I smile.
Twenty-four brand new hours are before me.
I vow to live fully in each moment and to look at all
beings with eyes of compassion."
— Thich Nhat Hanh

"IN LIFE, ONE HAS A CHOICE TO TAKE ONE OF TWO PATHS: TO WAIT FOR SOME SPECIAL DAY--OR TO MAKE EVERYDAY SPECIAL".

I AM GRATEFUL FOR...

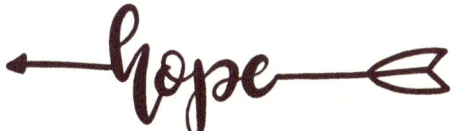

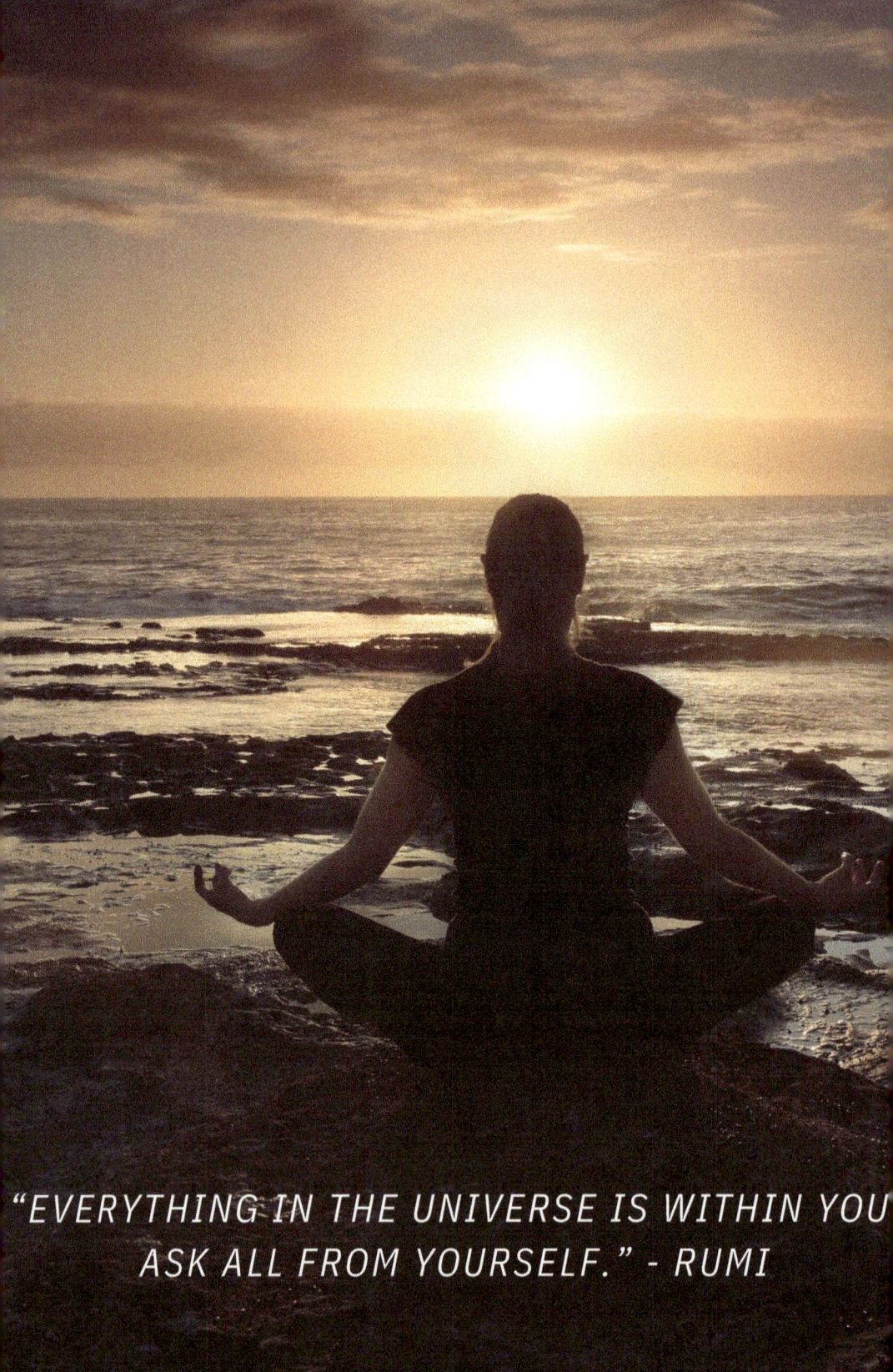

"FEELING GRATITUDE AND NOT EXPRESSING IT IS LIKE WRAPPING A PRESENT AND NOT GIVING IT." WILLIAM ARTHUR WARD

I AM GRATEFUL FOR...

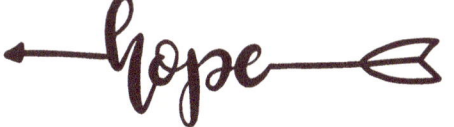

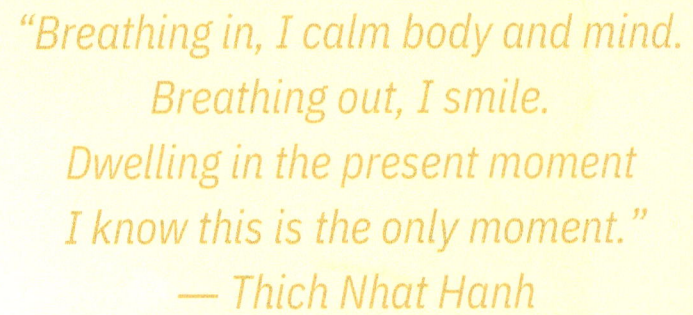

"Breathing in, I calm body and mind.
Breathing out, I smile.
Dwelling in the present moment
I know this is the only moment."
— Thich Nhat Hanh

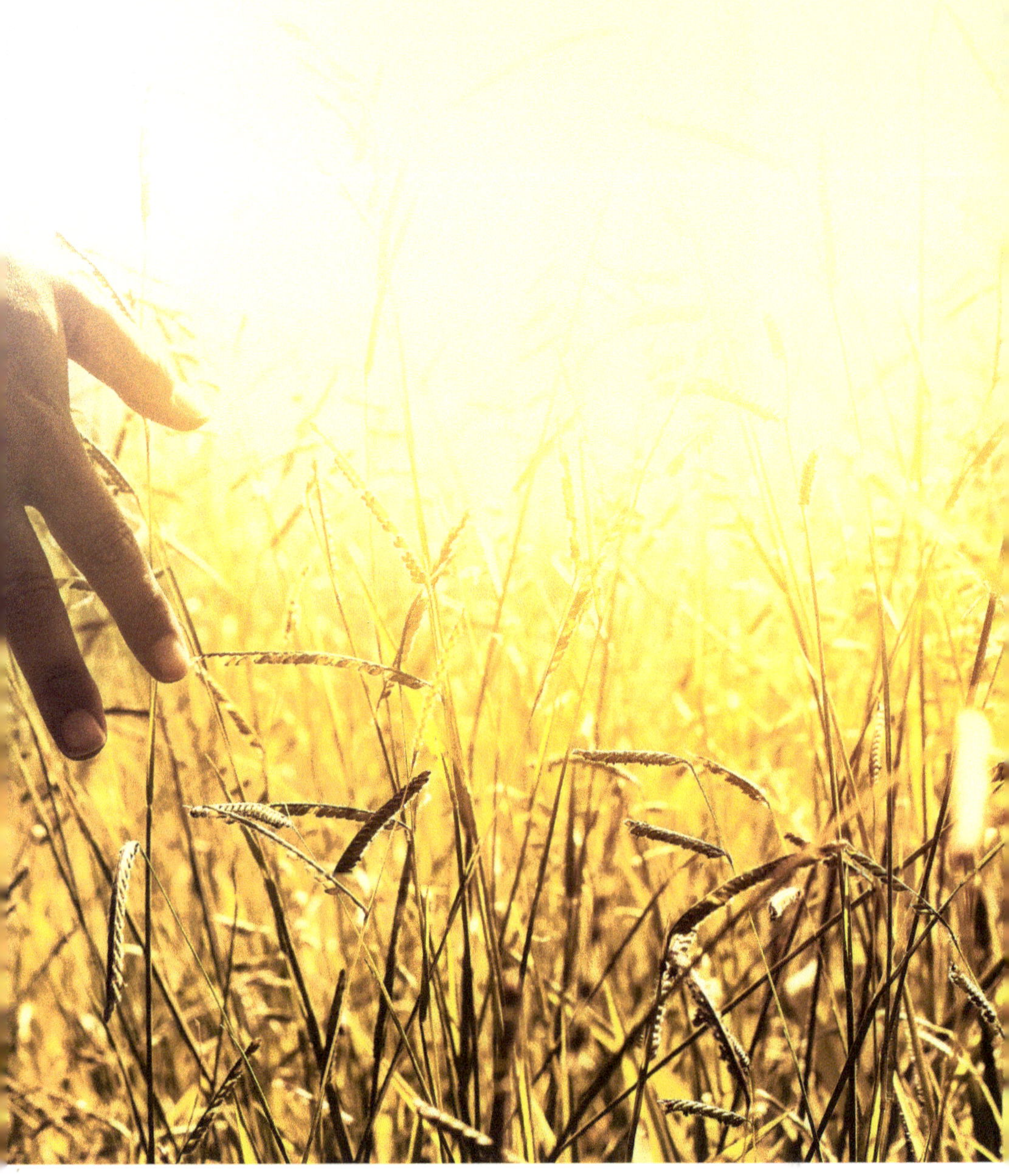

AN ATTITUDE OF GRATITUDE OPENS DOORS TO LIMITLESS POSSIBILITIES.

I AM GRATEFUL FOR...

hope

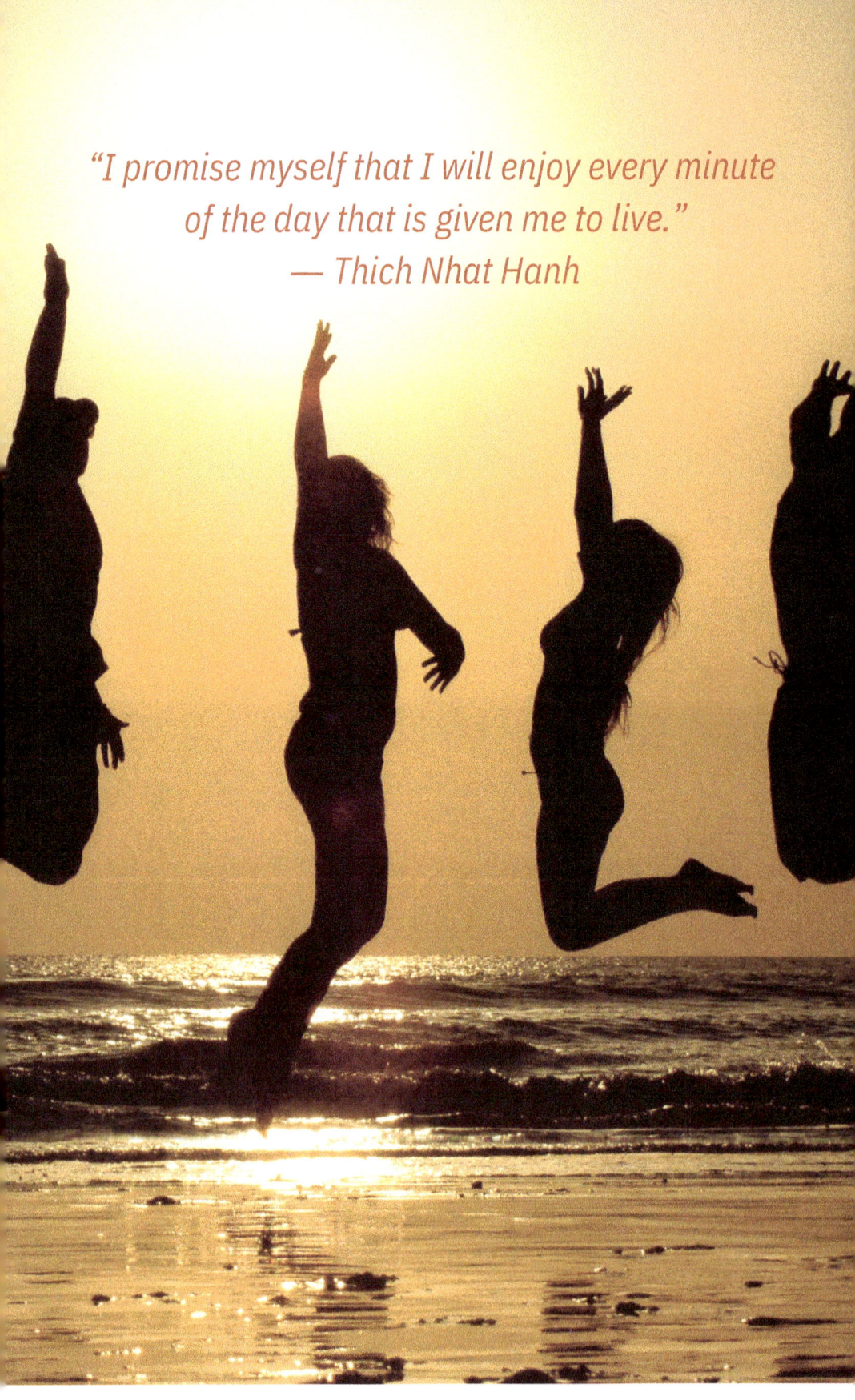

TODAY, I AM GRATEFUL FOR MY HEALTH. I AM INHALING VITALITY AND EXHALING TOXINS WITH EVERY BREATH. I AM THANKFUL FOR A HEALTHY MIND, BODY, AND SPIRIT.

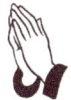

I AM GRATEFUL FOR...

hope

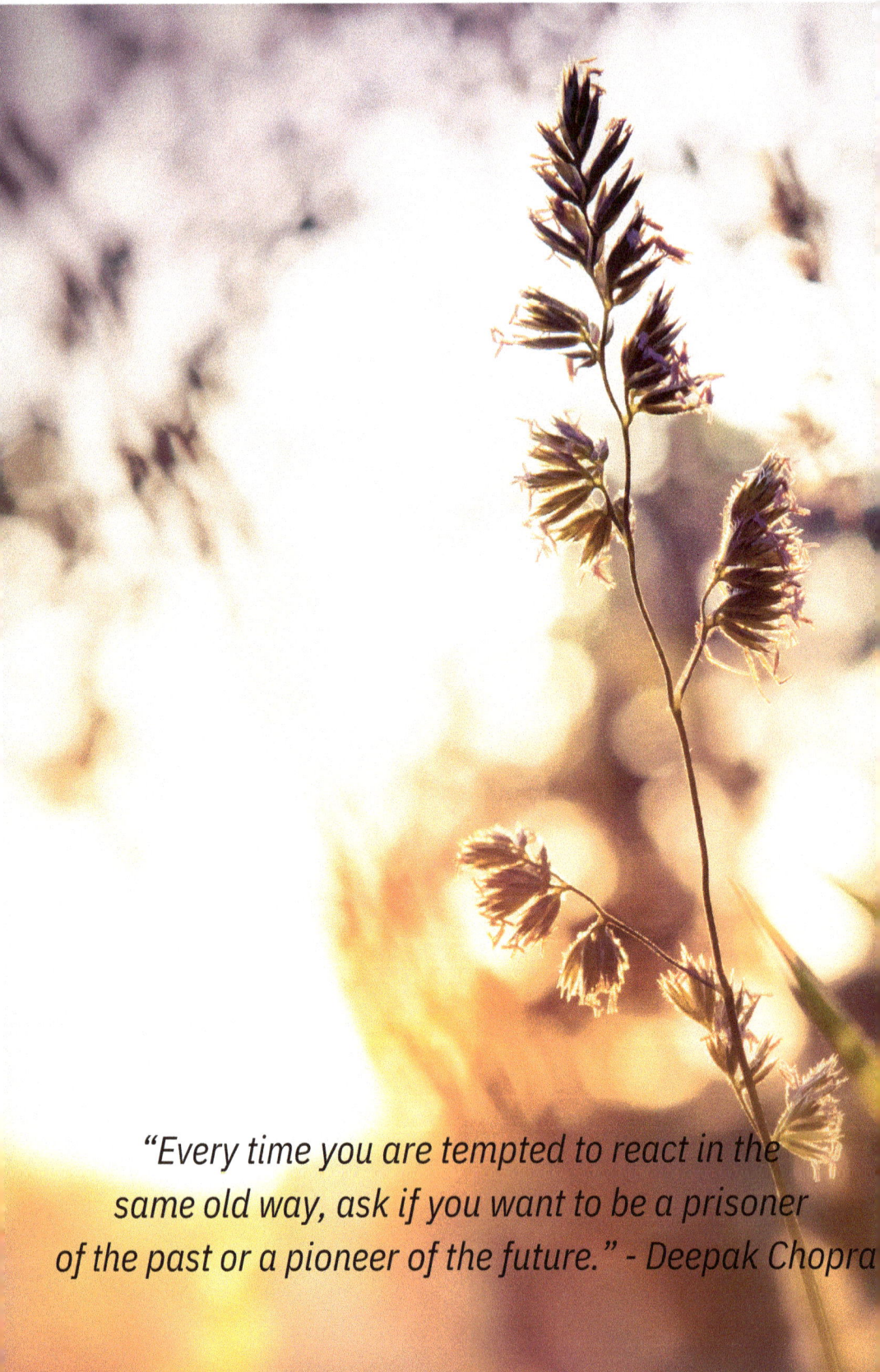

"REFLECT UPON YOUR PRESENT BLESSINGS, OF WHICH EVERY MAN HAS PLENTY; NOT ON YOUR PAST MISFORTUNES, OF WHICH ALL MEN HAVE SOME." CHARLES DICKENS

I AM GRATEFUL FOR...

hope

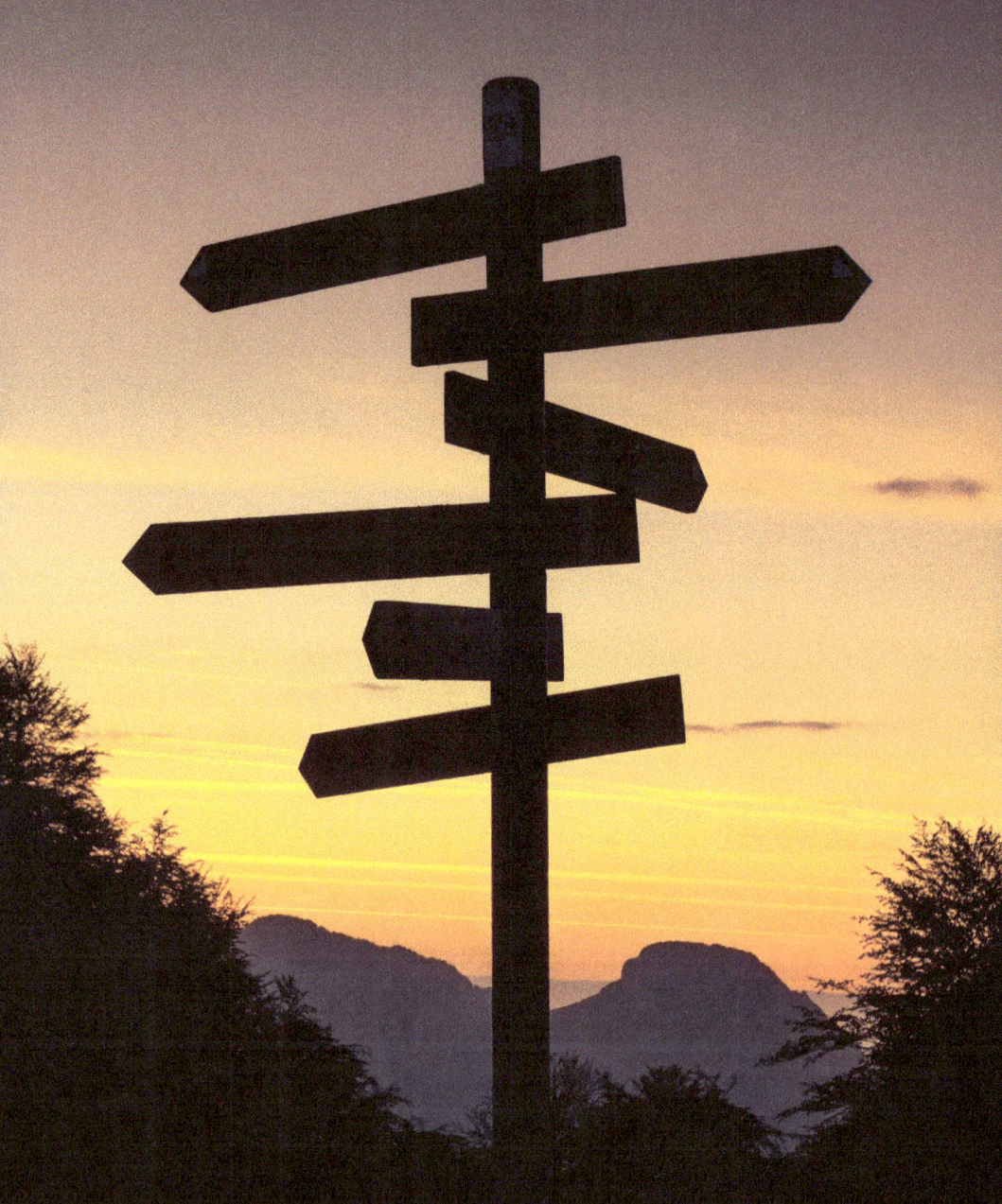

Your present choices create your future. Choose wisely.

"START EACH DAY WITH A POSITIVE THOUGHT AND A GRATEFUL HEART." —ROY T. BENNETT,

I AM GRATEFUL FOR...

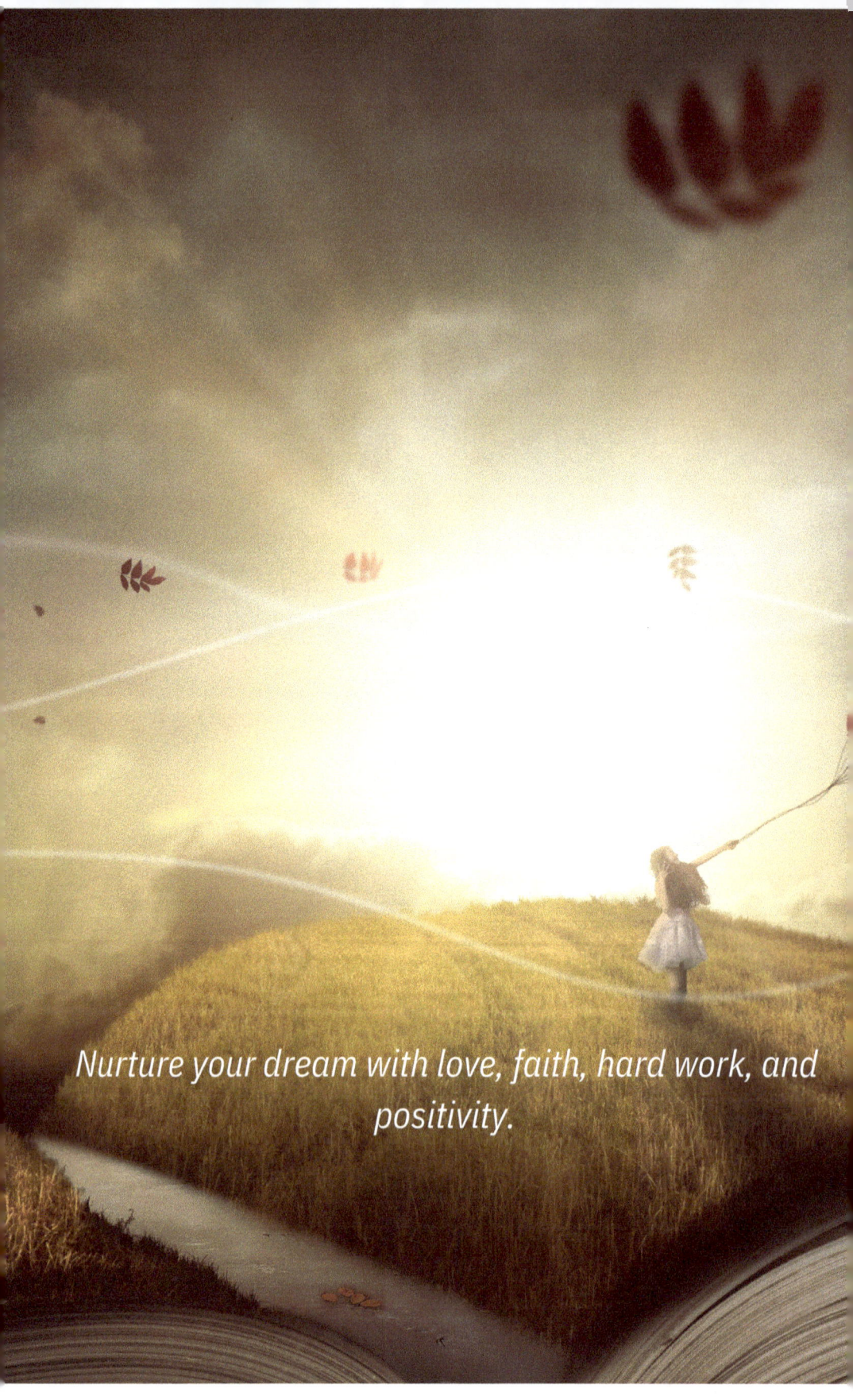
Nurture your dream with love, faith, hard work, and positivity.

BE GRATEFUL FOR WHAT YOU CURRENTLY HAVE WHILE YOU CHASE YOUR DREAMS, IF YOU CANNOT APPRECIATE WHAT YOU HAVE, HOW WILL YOU VALUE WHAT YOU GET?

I AM GRATEFUL FOR...

hope

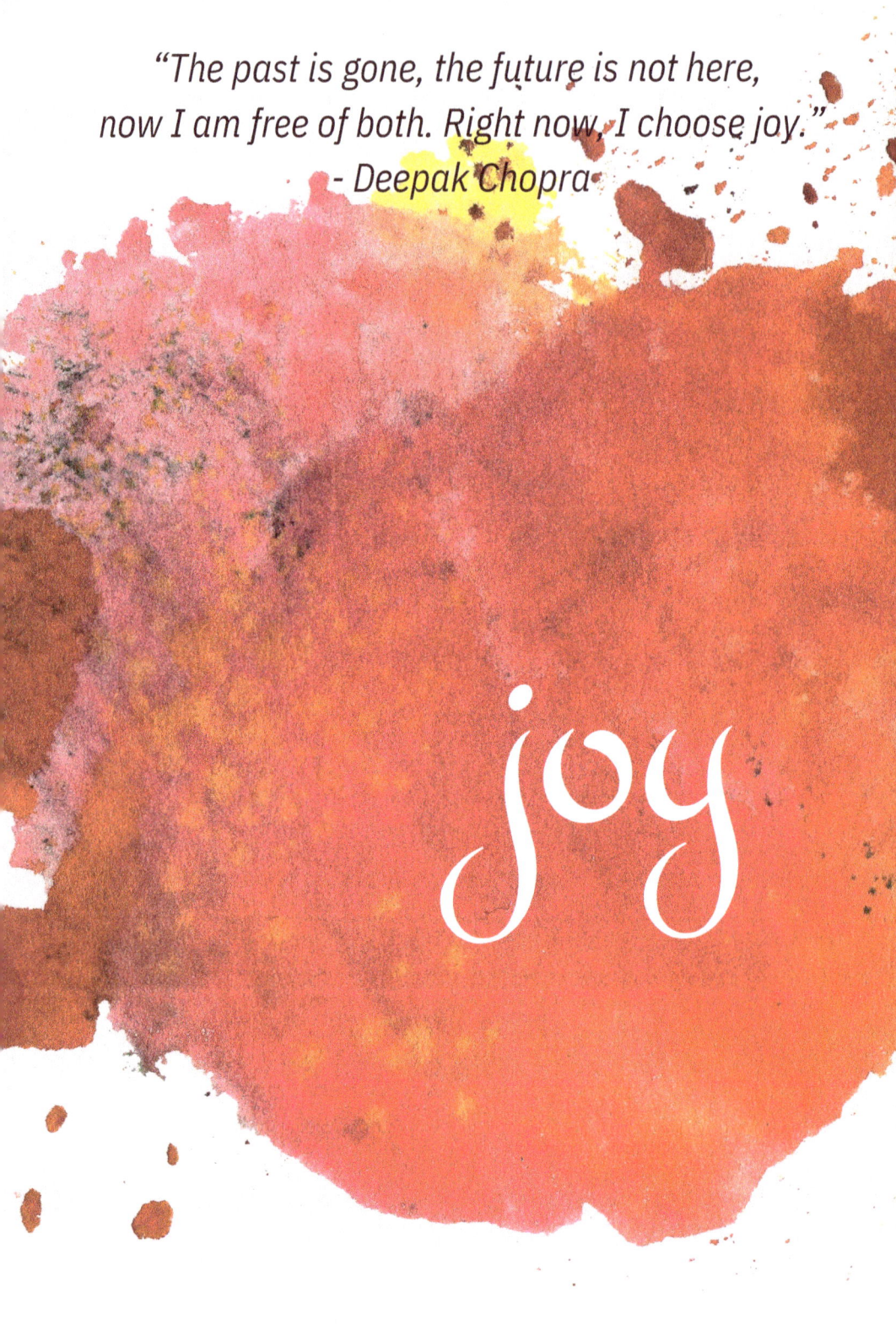

"DEVELOPING AN ATTITUDE OF GRATITUDE IS NOT A ROCKET SCIENCE. IT JUST TAKES A CHANGE OF MINDSET."

I AM GRATEFUL FOR...

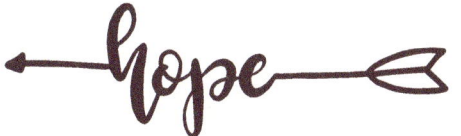

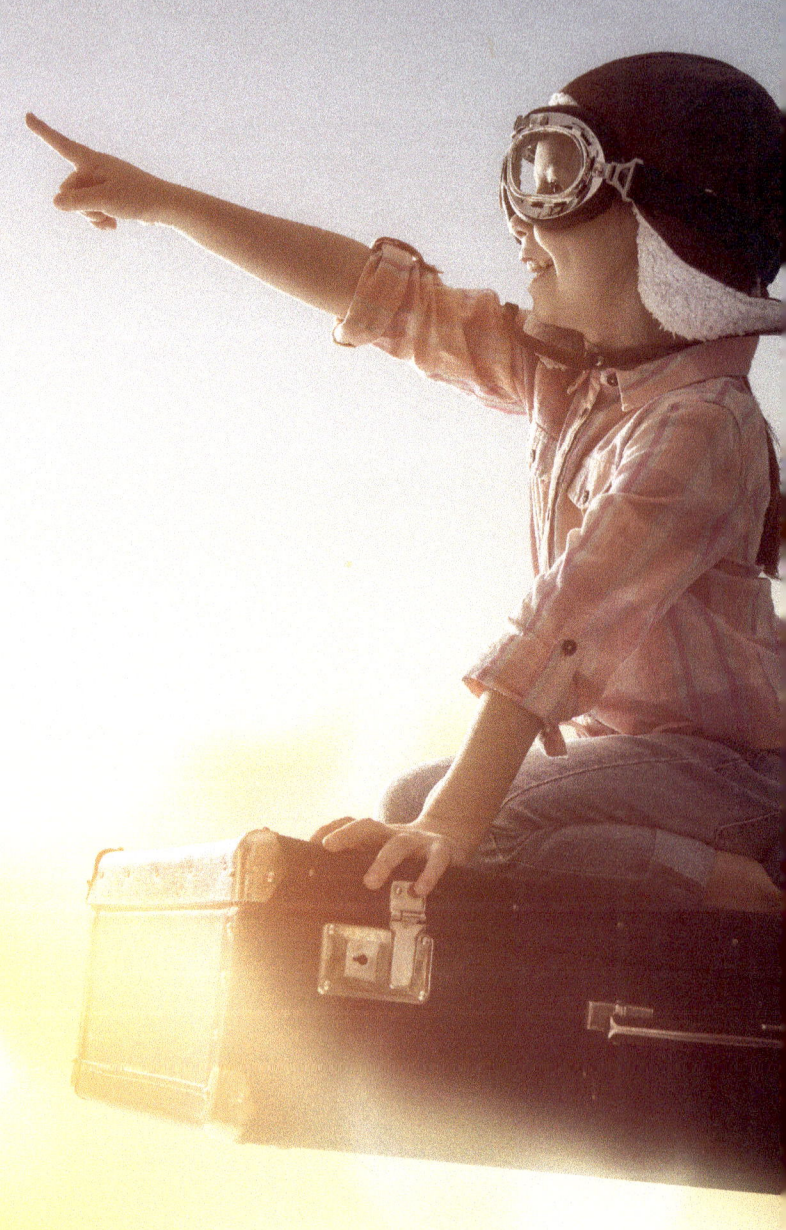

Chase your dreams with every ounce of energy you have because Impossible = I M Possible

"GRATITDUE = ENDORPHINS - HAPPINESS."

I AM GRATEFUL FOR...

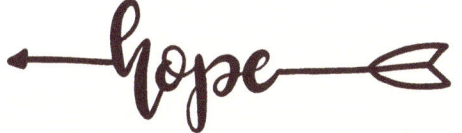

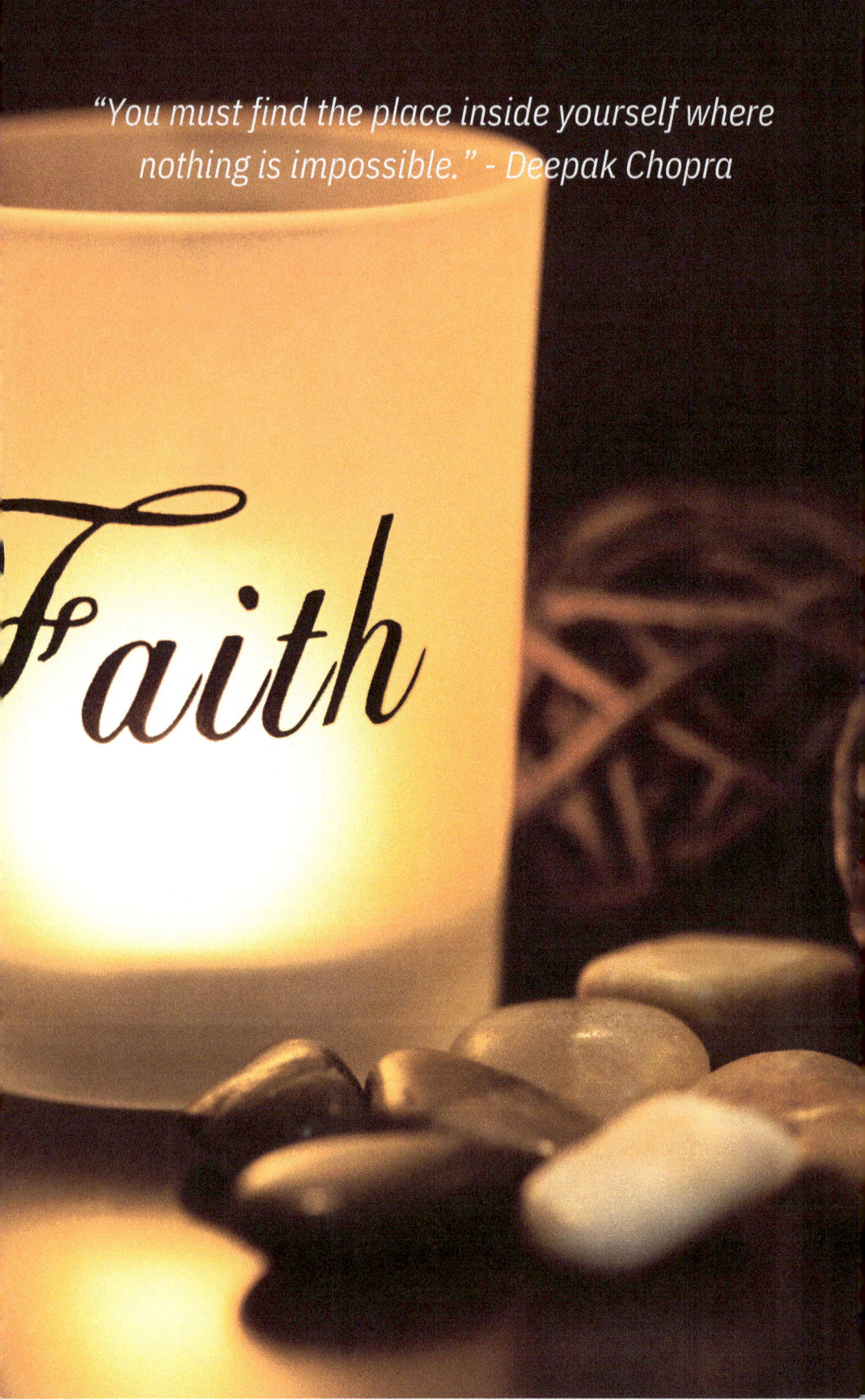

LIFE IS A MIRACLE. COUNT YOUR BLESSINGS

I AM GRATEFUL FOR...

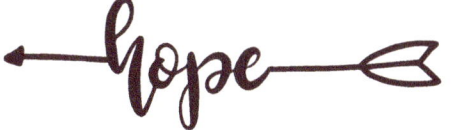

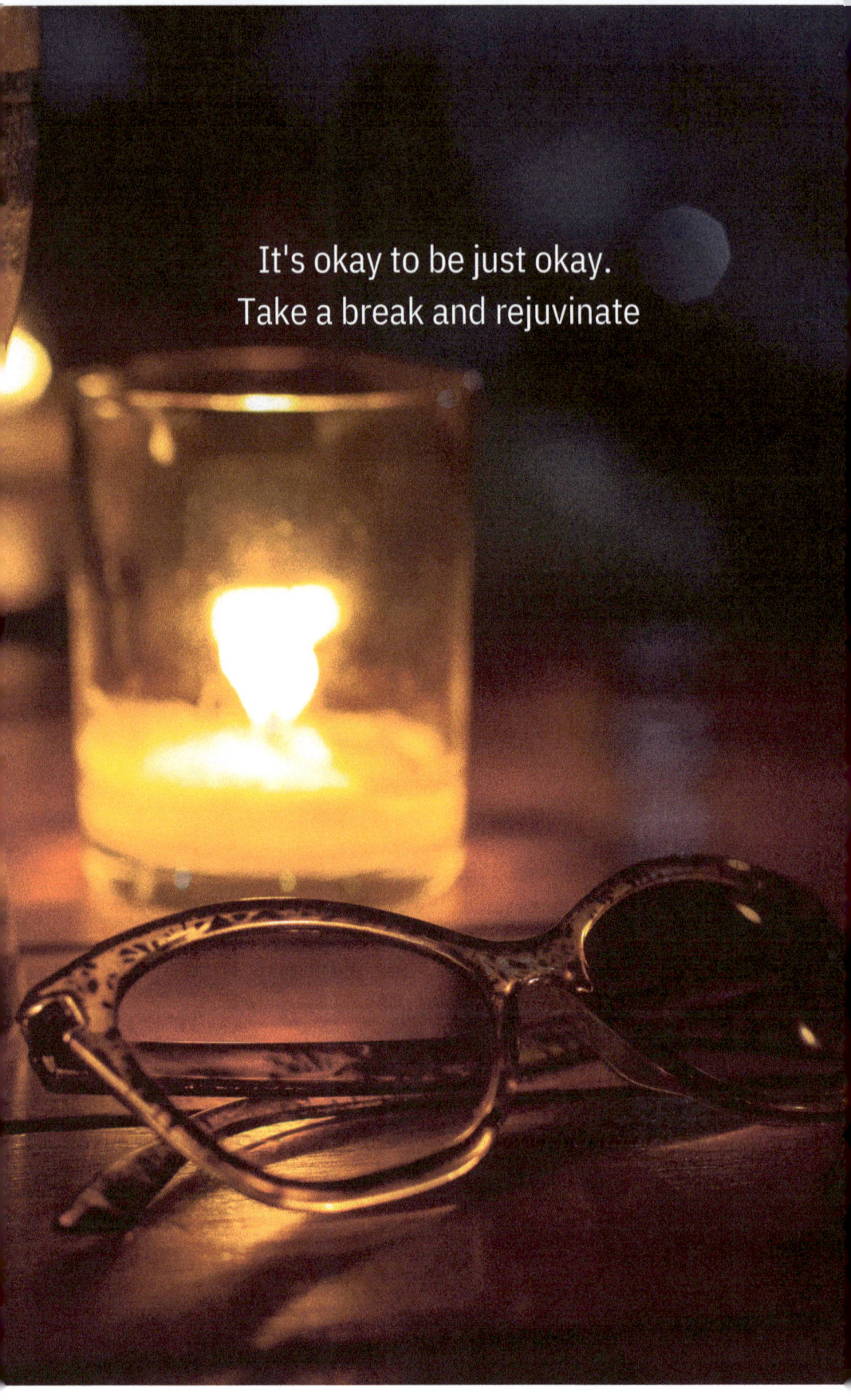

BE GRATEFUL FOR THE SUNSHINE AND BUTTERFLIES. BE GRATEFUL FOR THE BEES AND BIRDS. BE GRATEFUL FOR THE HEALING POWER OF NATURE.

I AM GRATEFUL FOR...

hope

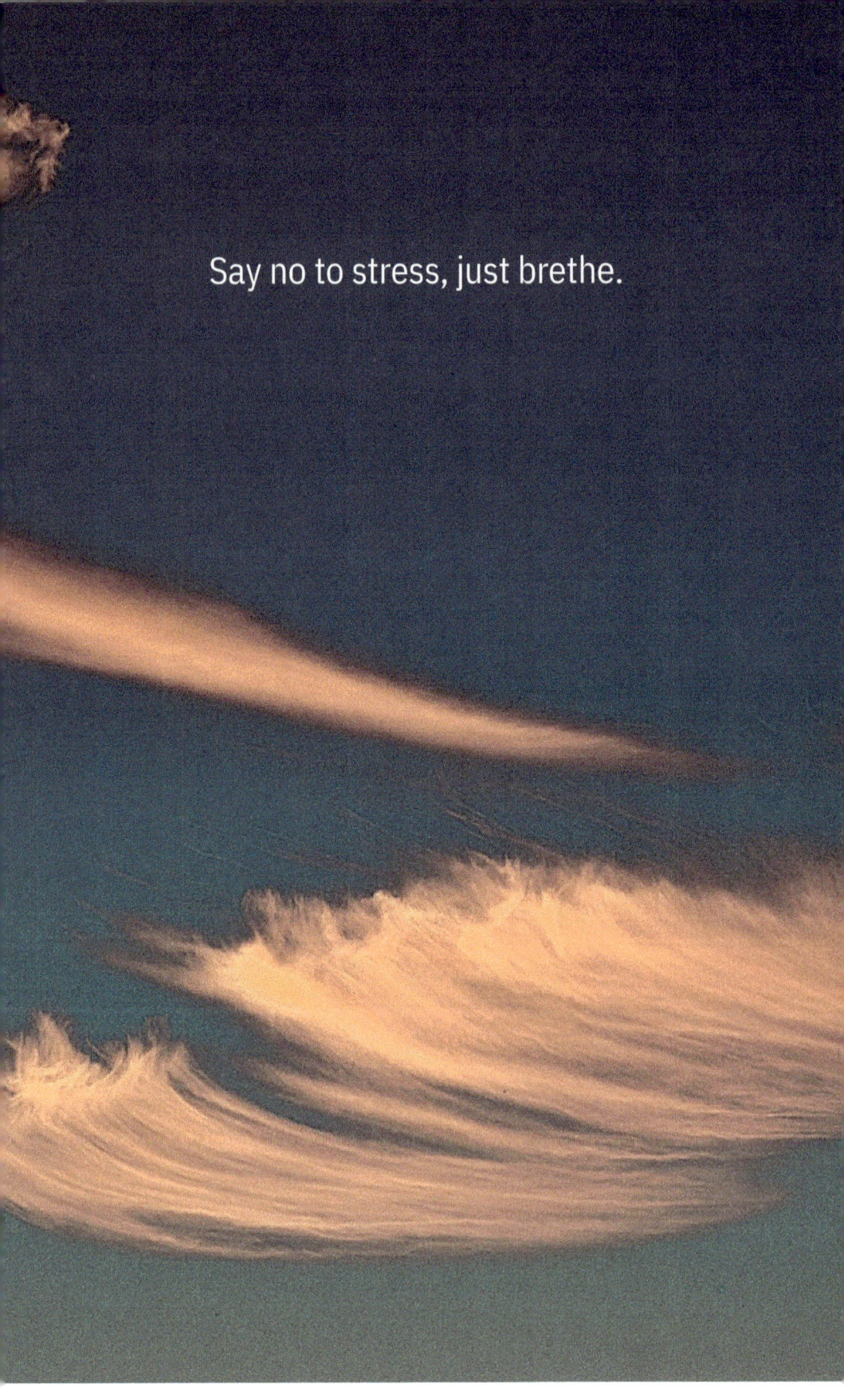

TODAY I AM GRATEFUL FOR PERFECT HEALTH. MY BODY HAS AN AMAZING ABILITY TO HEAL ITSELF. I AM BLESSED.

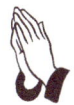

I AM GRATEFUL FOR...

hope

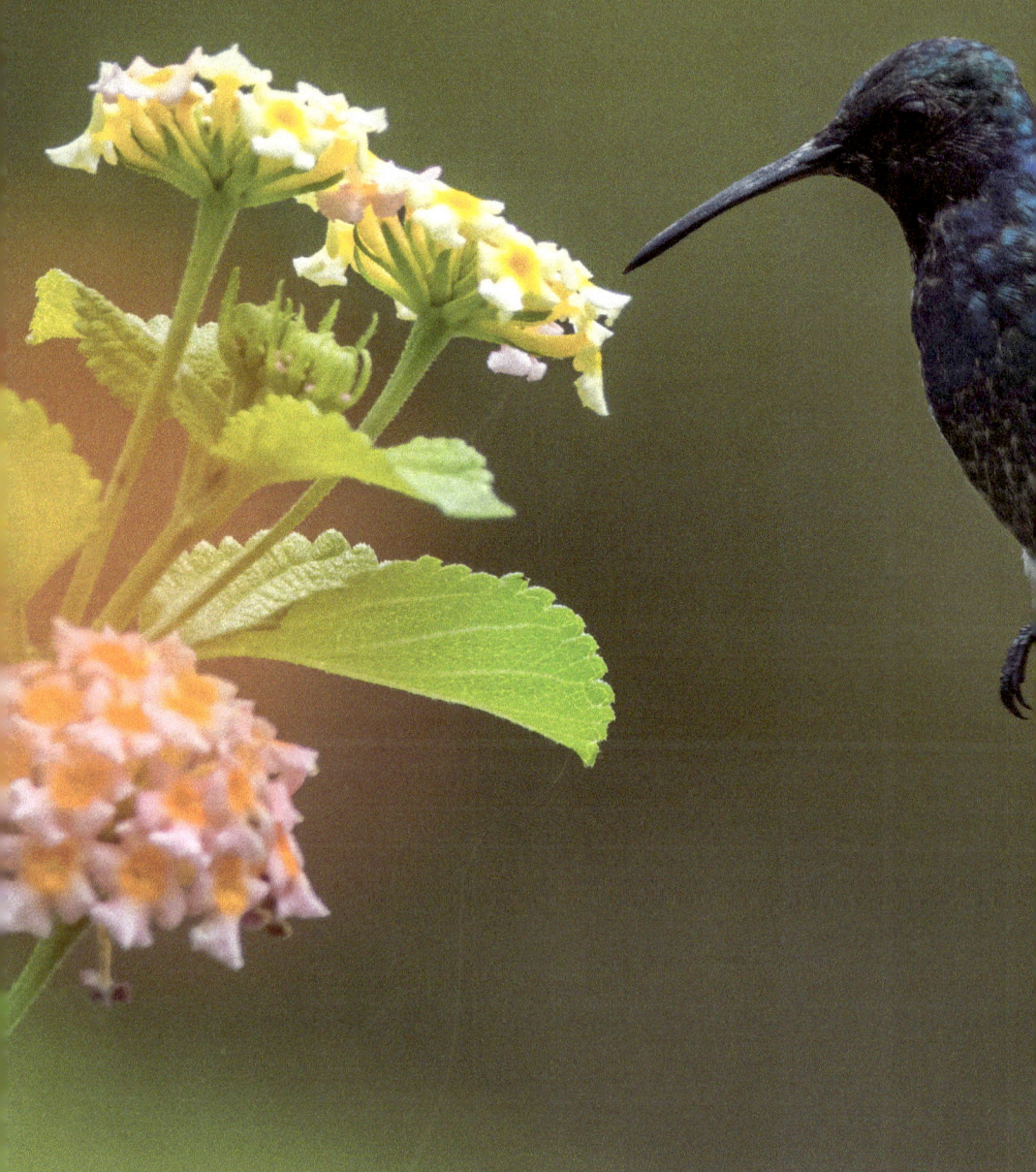

We carry inside us the wonders we seek outside us - Rumi

I AM GRATEFUL THAT I AM ATTRACTING ABUNDANCE IN MY LIFE EFFORTLESSLY.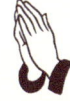

I AM GRATEFUL FOR...

hope

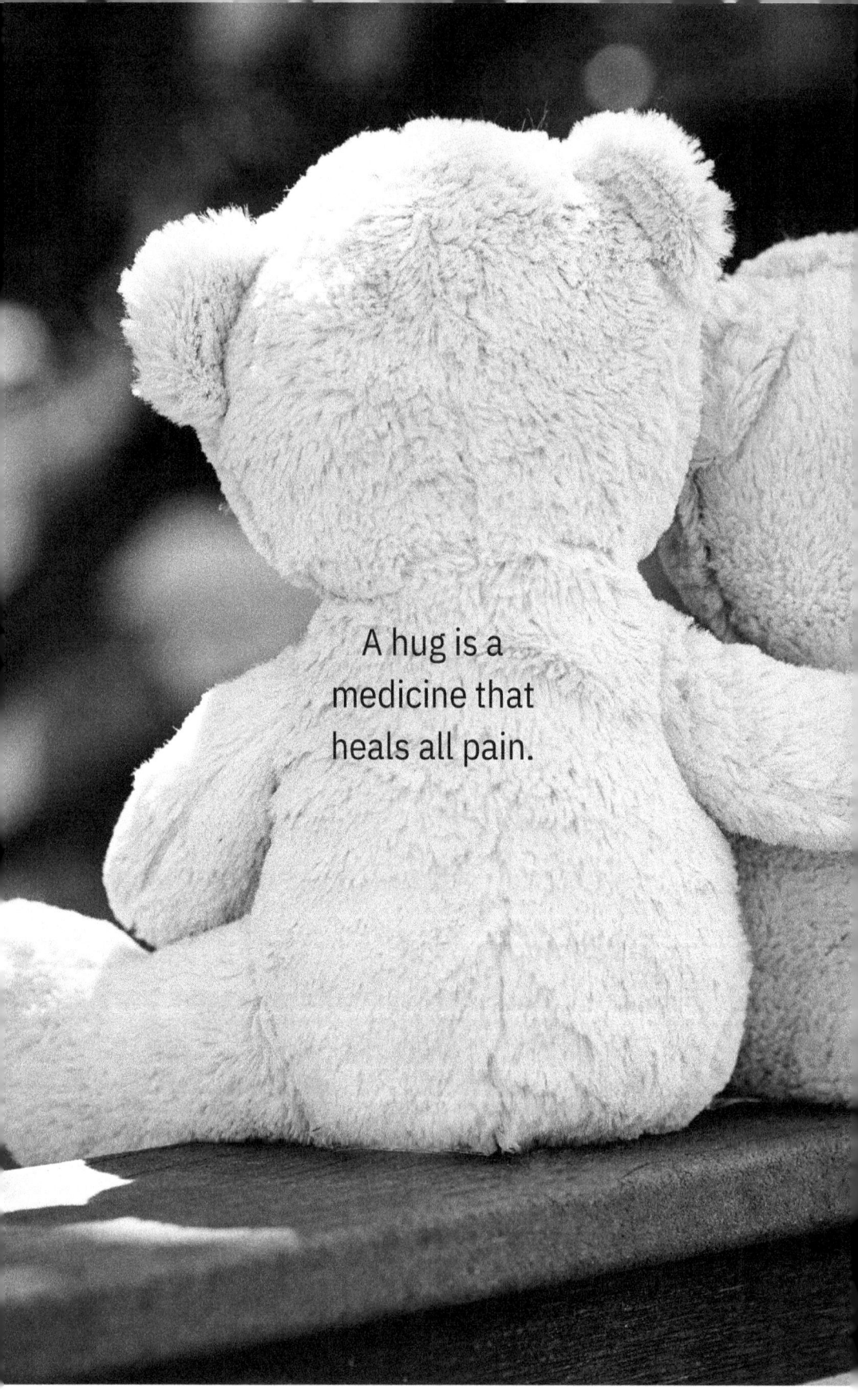

I AM THANKFUL AND THAT'S WHY I AM HAPPY. IT'S NOT THE OTHER WAY AROUND.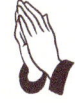

I AM GRATEFUL FOR...

Repeat after me
"I love and accept myself unconditionally."

I AM GRATEFUL FOR EVERYTHING I HAVE AND I AM ATTRACTING MORE PROSPERITY.

I AM GRATEFUL FOR...

hope

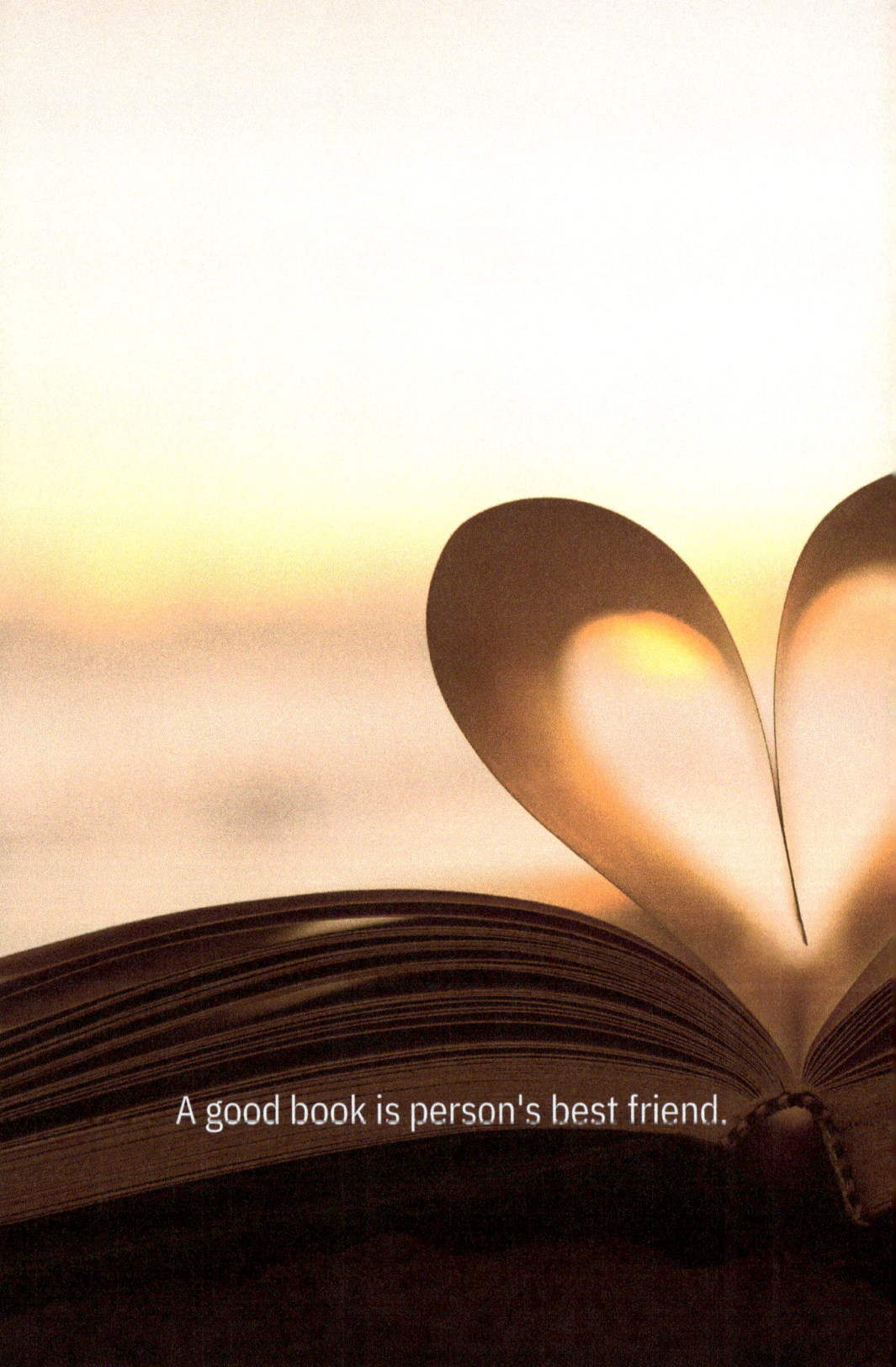

GRATITUDE CAN TAKE YOU FROM LACK TO ABUDANCE

I AM GRATEFUL FOR...

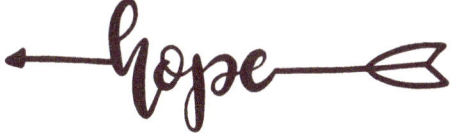

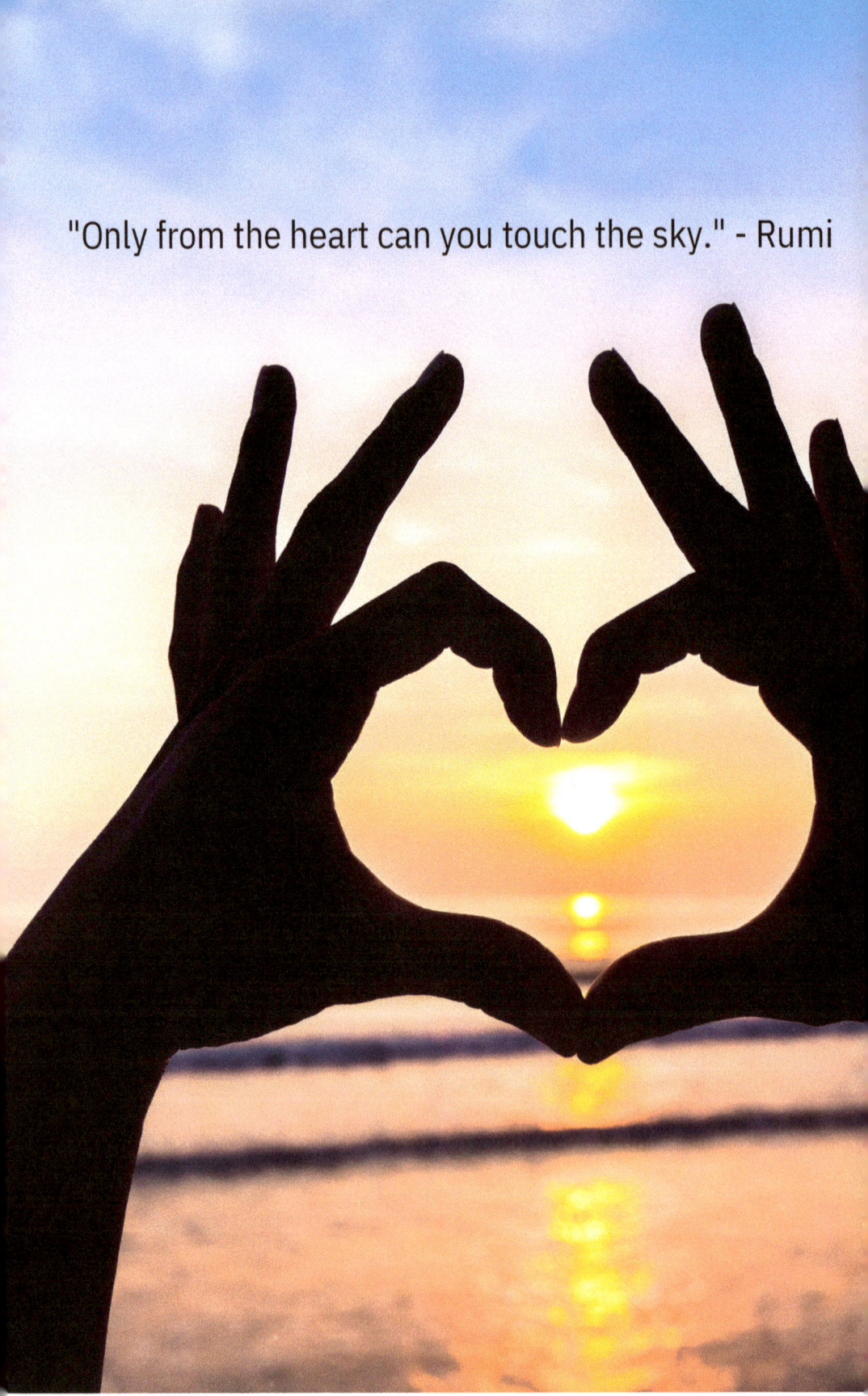

AN ATTITUDE OF GRATITUDE WILL TURN YOUR DREAMS INTO REALITY.

I AM GRATEFUL FOR...

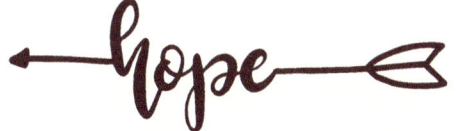

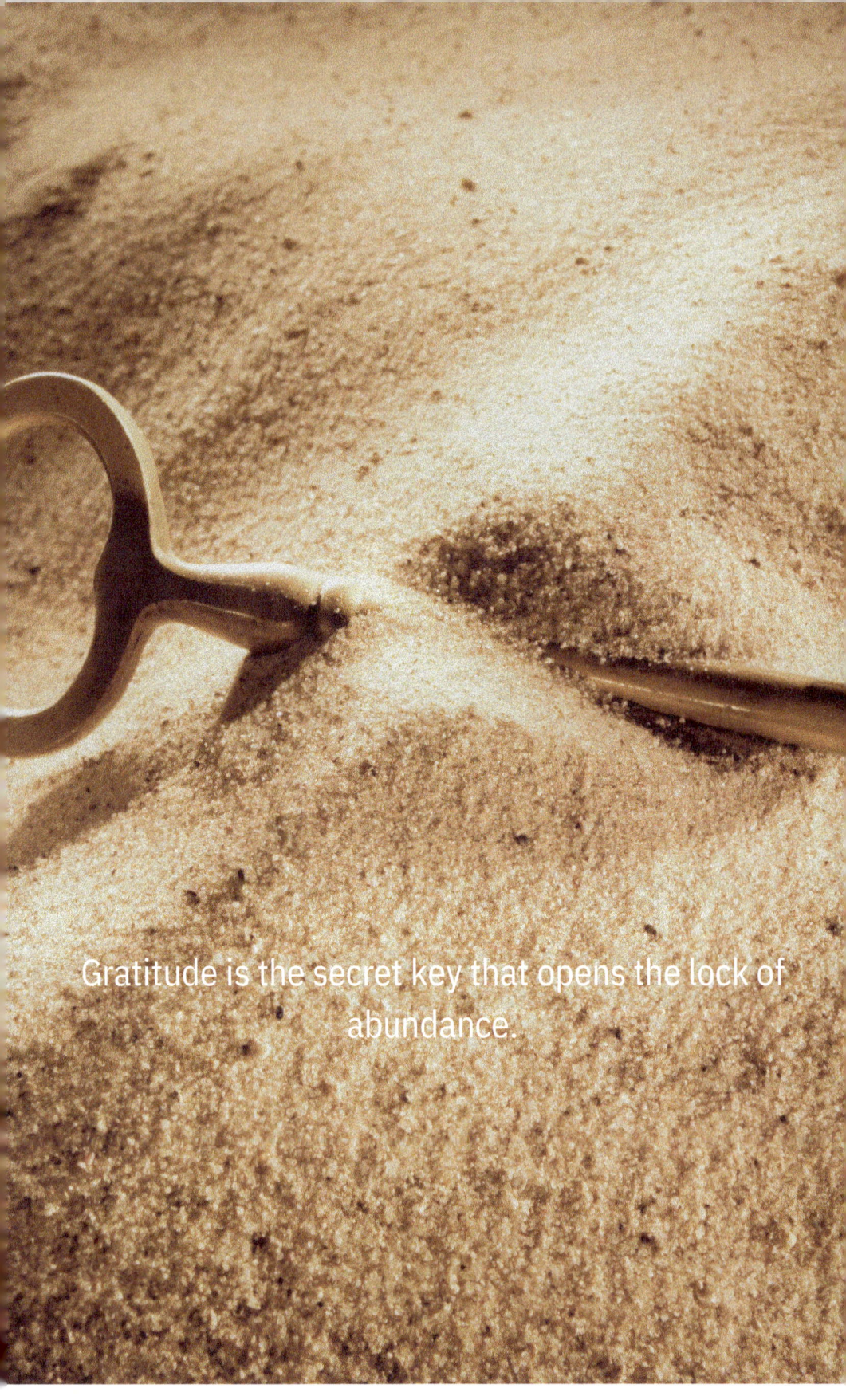

AN ATTITUDE OF GRATITUDE PRESENTS LIMITLESS OPPORTUNITIES.

TODAY I AM GRATEFUL FOR...

hope

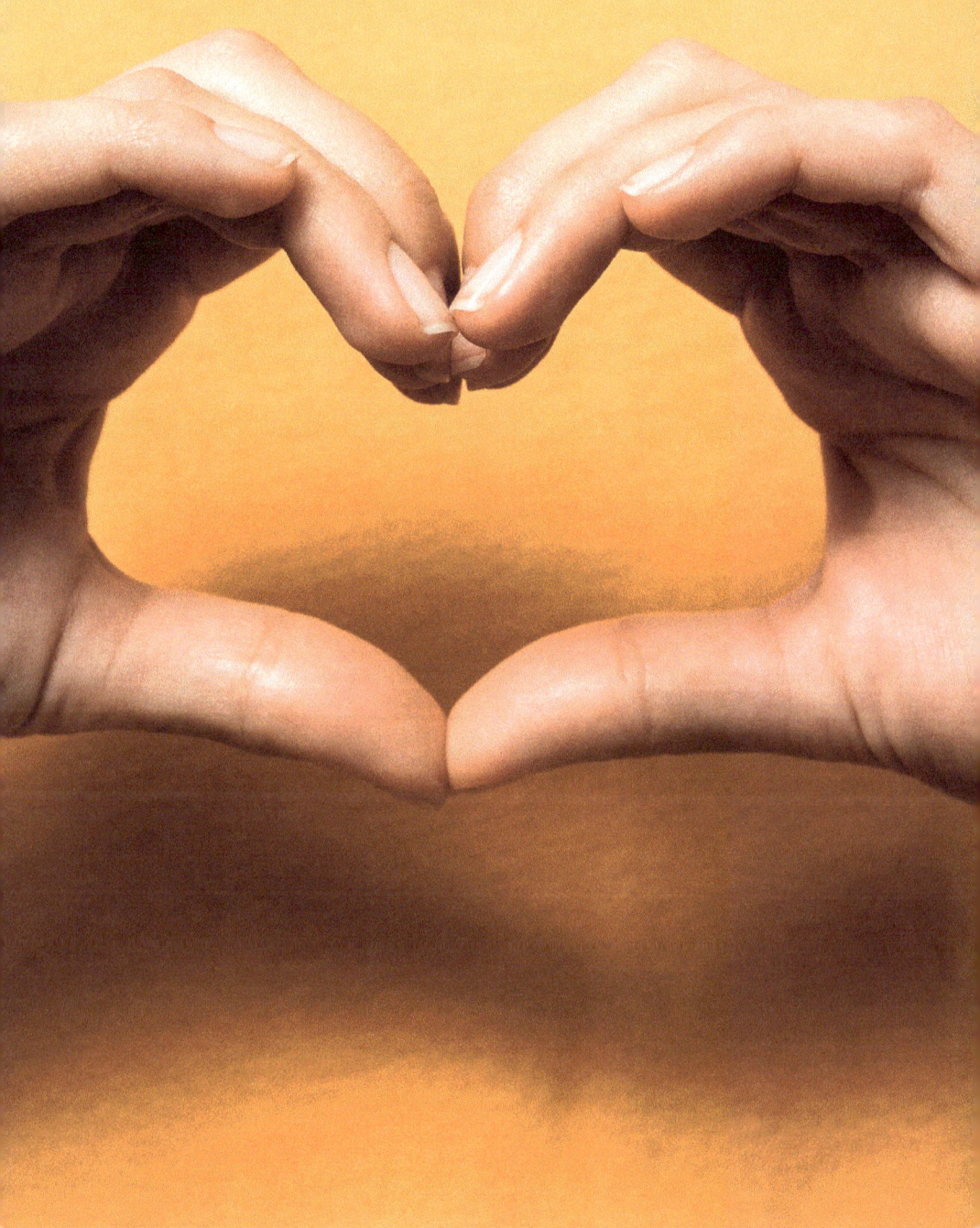

Self-acceptance and self-love are two keys that opens the lock to happiness.

AN ATTITUDE OF GRATITUDE IS AN OPPORTUNITY TO CHANGE YOUR LIFE.

I AM GRATEFUL FOR...

hope

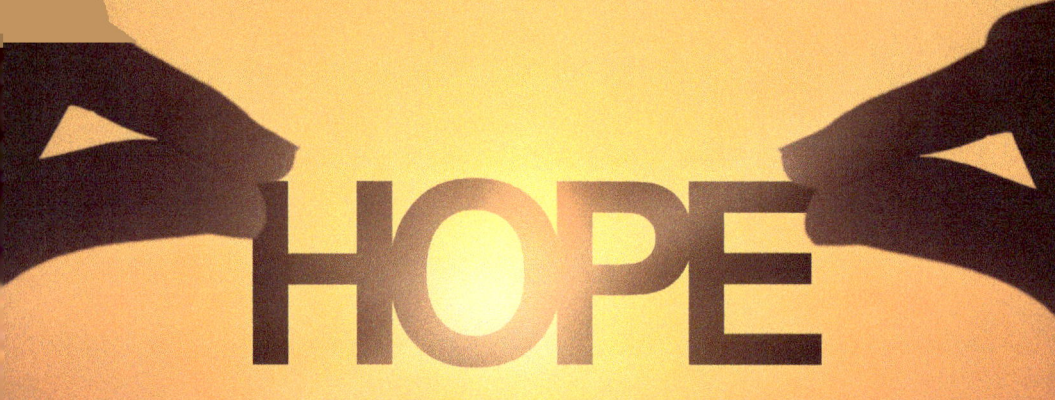

CHANGE YOUR ATTITUDE, CHANGE YOUR HEALTH.

I AM GRATEFUL FOR...

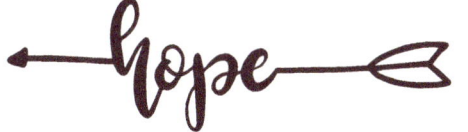

Some days, you just have to take it easy, hunker down, and let the storm pass by.

EVERY DAY IS A BLANK SLATE FOR YOU TO WRITE YOUR OWN DESTINY. YOUR ACTIONS CREATE YOUR FUTURE. ACT WISELY.

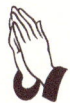

I AM GRATEFUL FOR...

hope

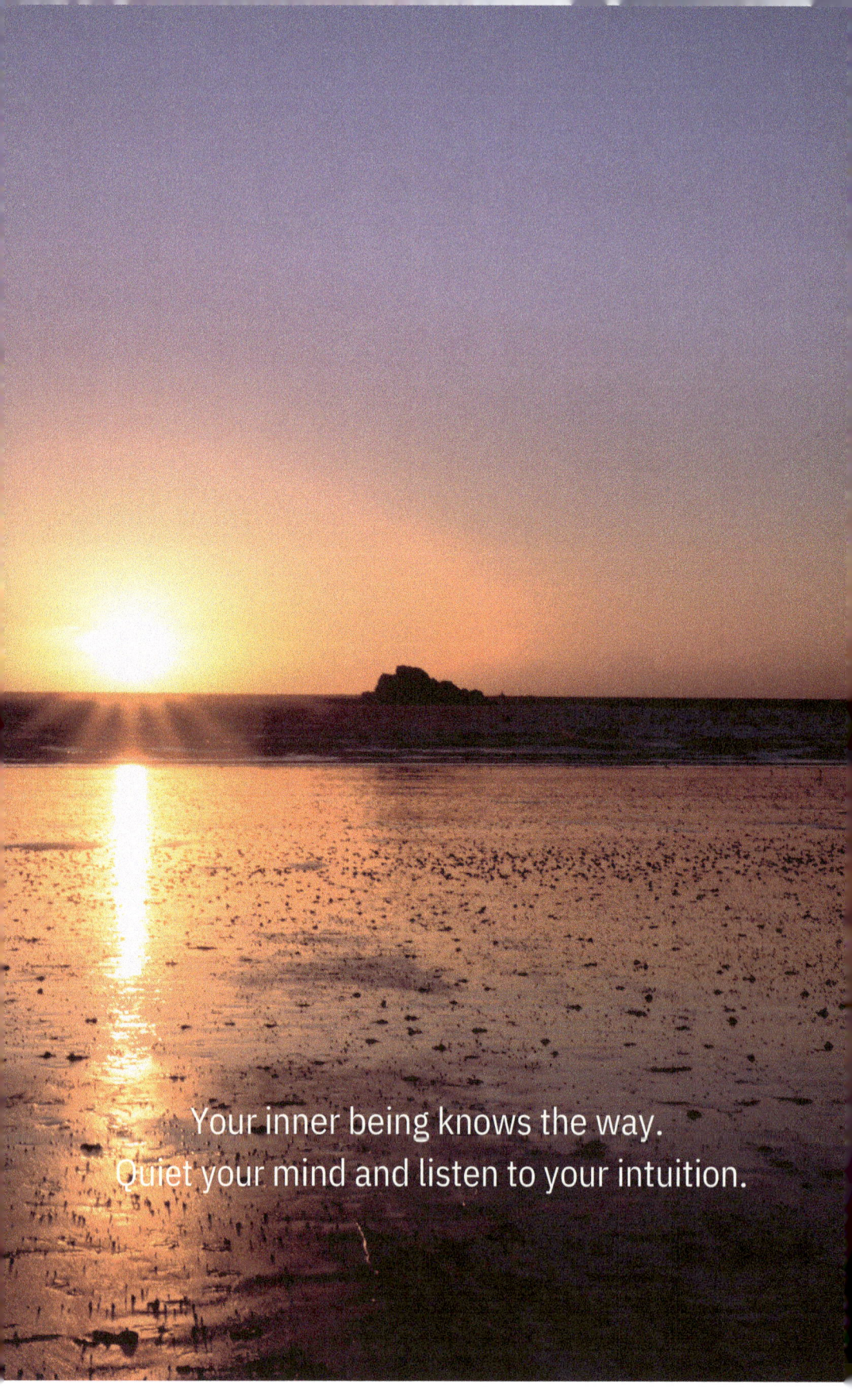

LIFE IS FULL OF MIRACLES AND THEY ONLY HAPPEN WHEN WE APPRECIATE WHAT WE HAVE.

I AM GRATEFUL FOR...

hope

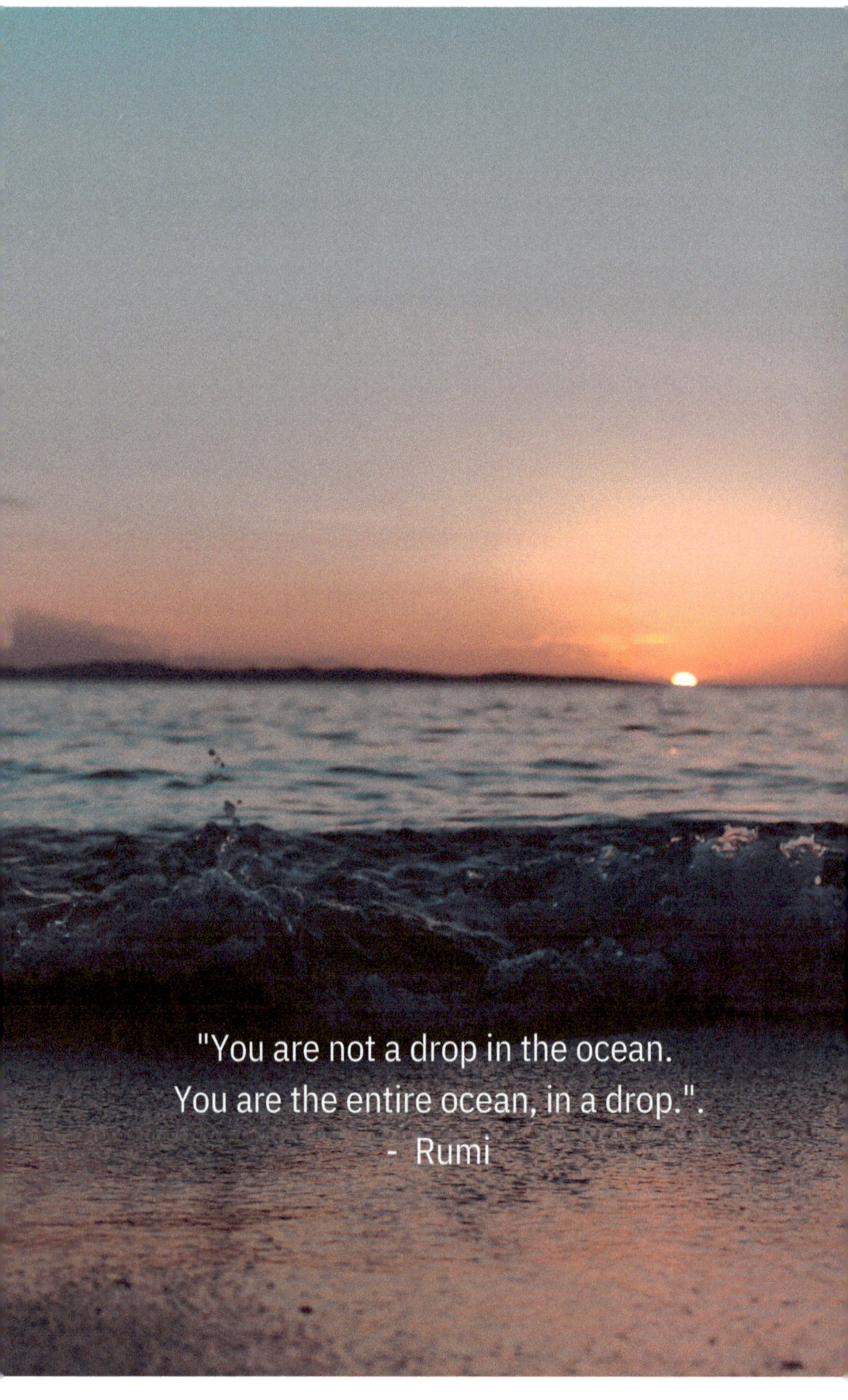

BE A BLESSING IN SOMEONE'S LIFE AND YOU WILL ATTAIN HAPPINESS.

I AM GRATEFUL FOR...

hope

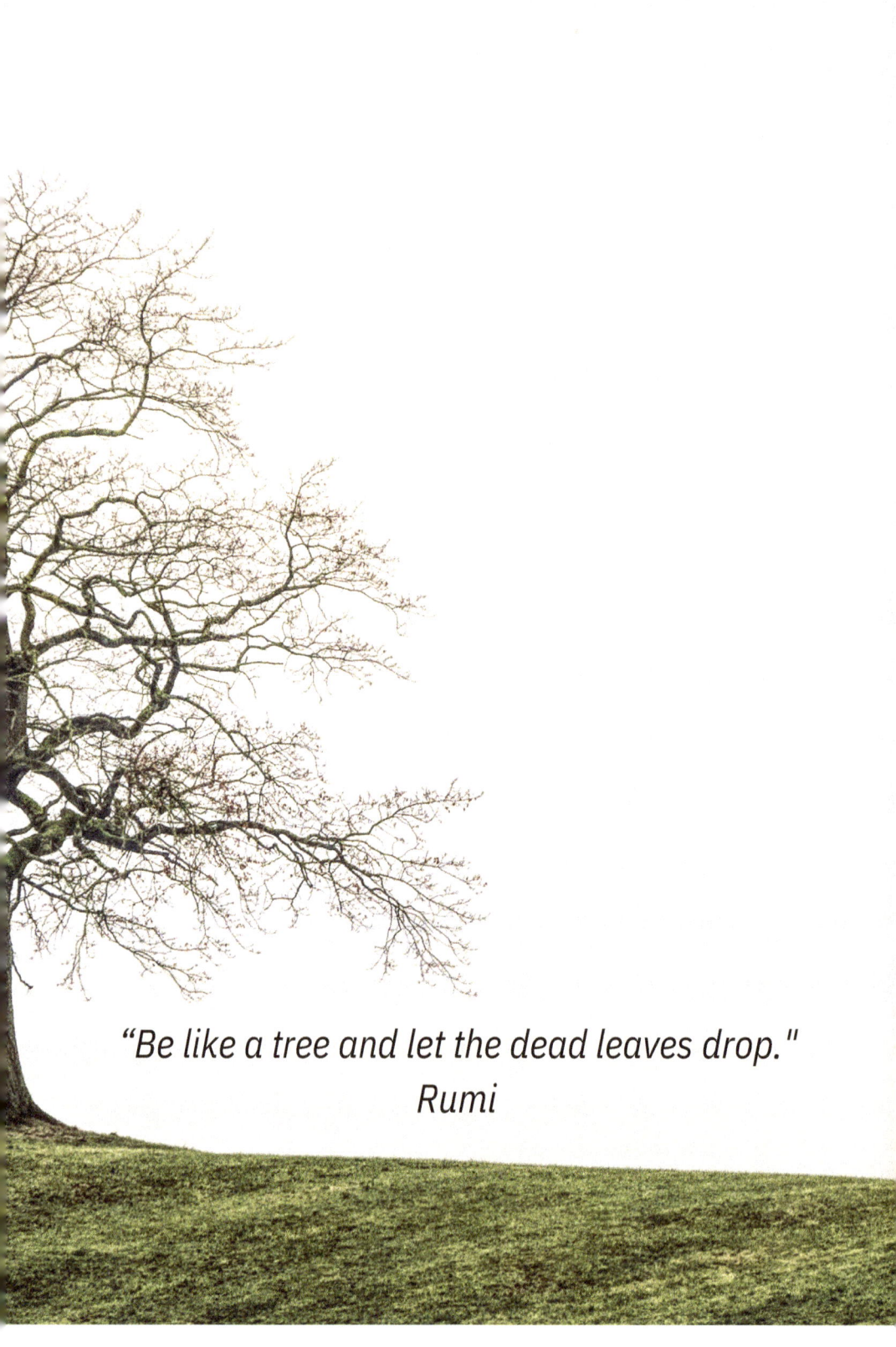
"Be like a tree and let the dead leaves drop."
Rumi

I AM GRATEFUL FOR THE MISTAKES I HAVE MADE BECAUSE THEY MADE ME WISER.

I AM GRATEFUL FOR...

hope

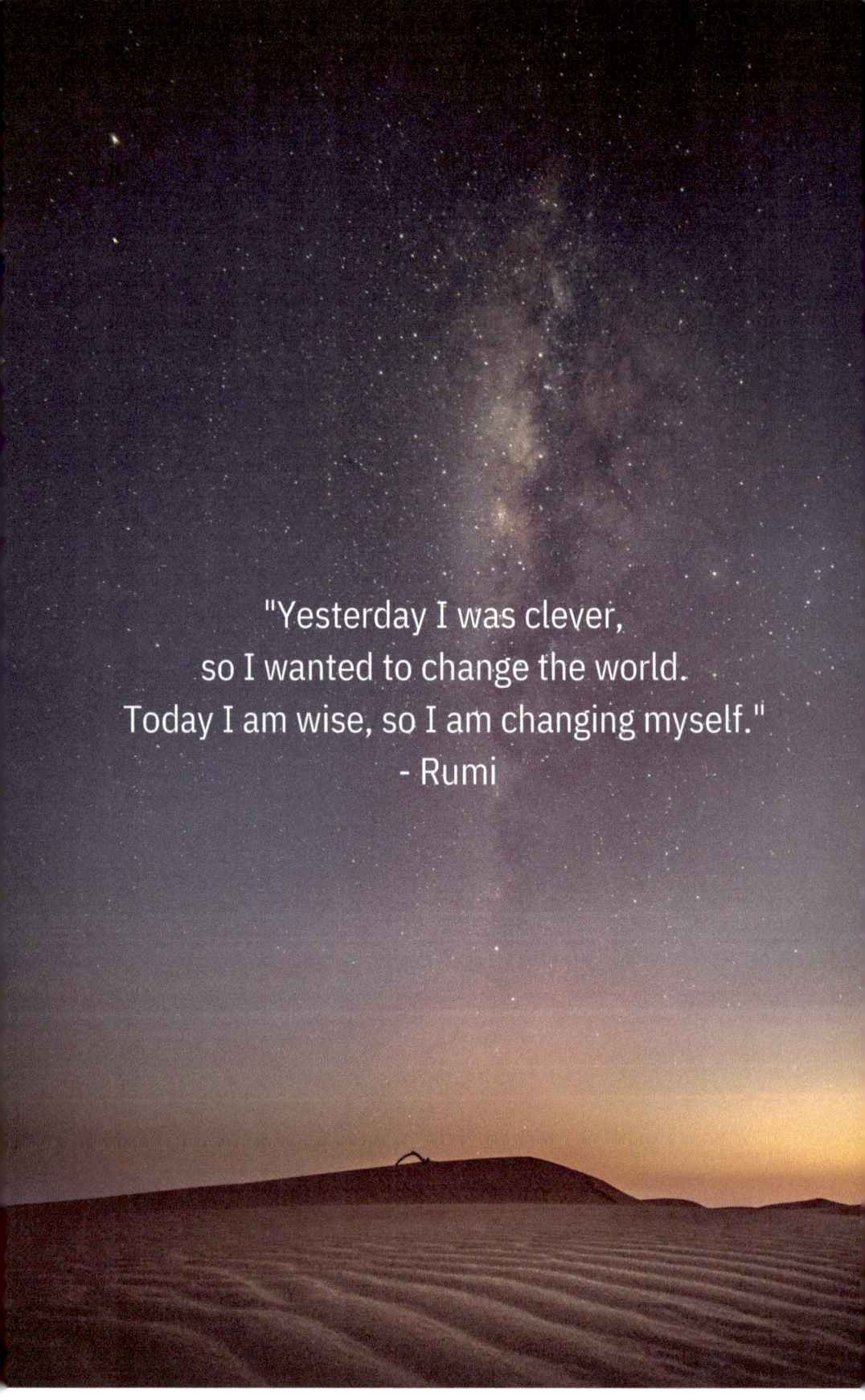

GRATITUDE IS A UNIVERSAL LANGUAGE. IT IS A PRAYER THAT IS ALWAYS ANSWERED.

I AM GRATEFUL FOR...

hope

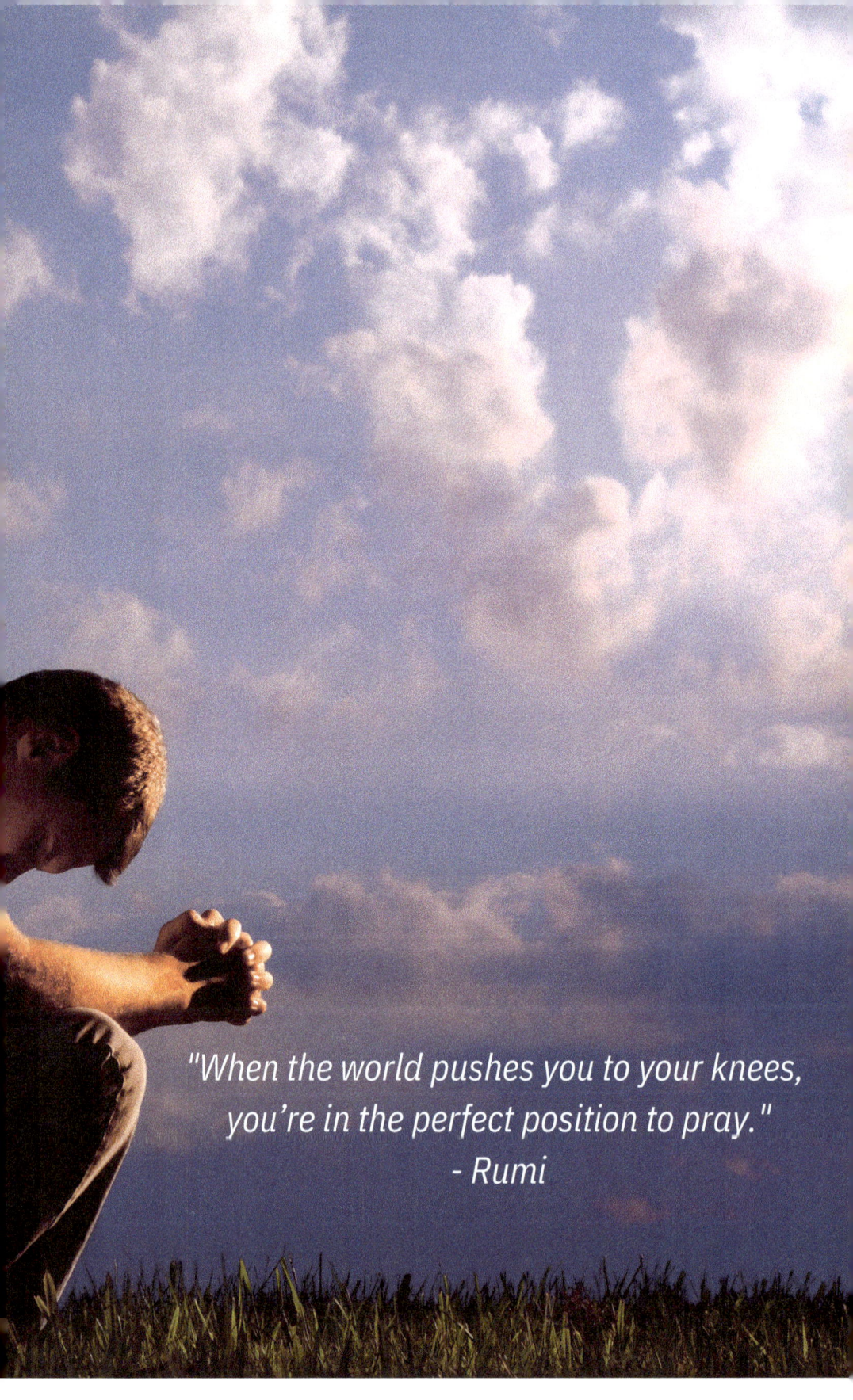

AN ATTITUDE OF GRATITUDE HAS AN AMAZING POWER TO CREATE MIRACLES THAT ARE BEYOND THE LOGICAL MIND.

I AM GRATEFUL FOR...

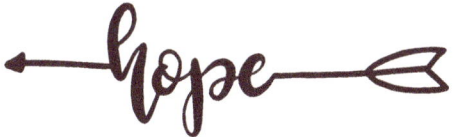

"Only when I love and accept myself unconditionally, I can love and accept others for what they are."

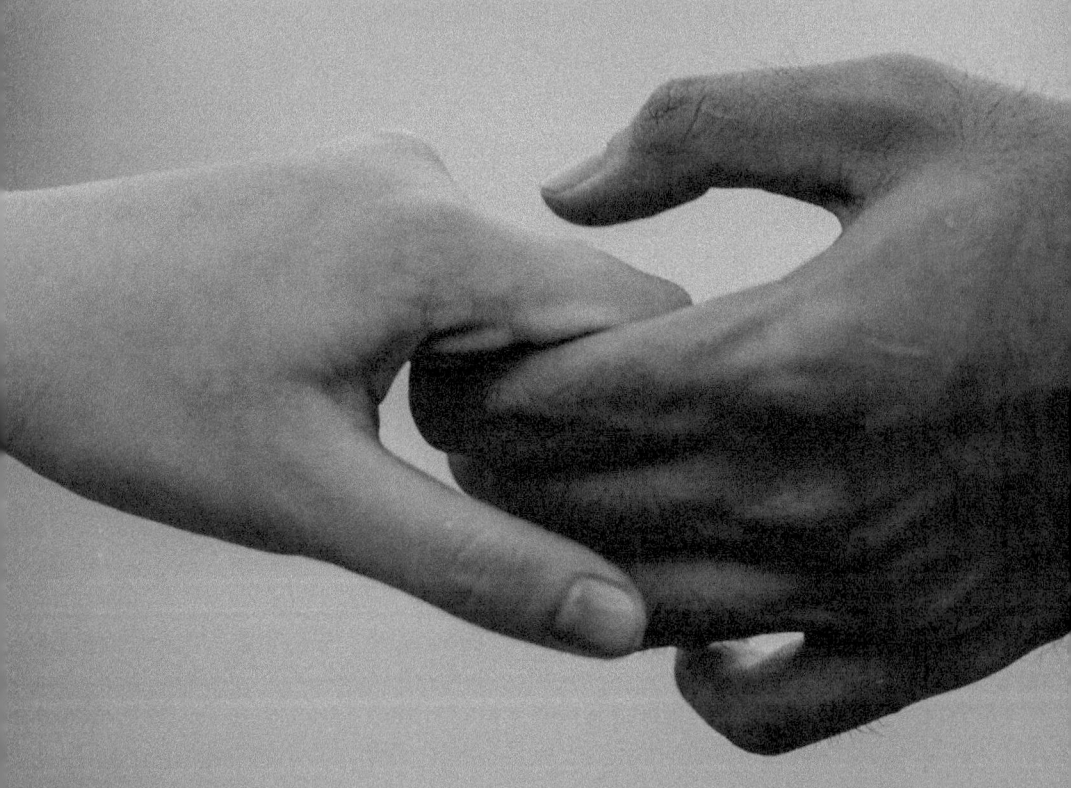

I AM GRATEFUL FOR WHAT I HAVE AND THAT IS WHY I AM BLESSED WITH PROSPERITY.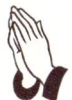

I AM GRATEFUL FOR...

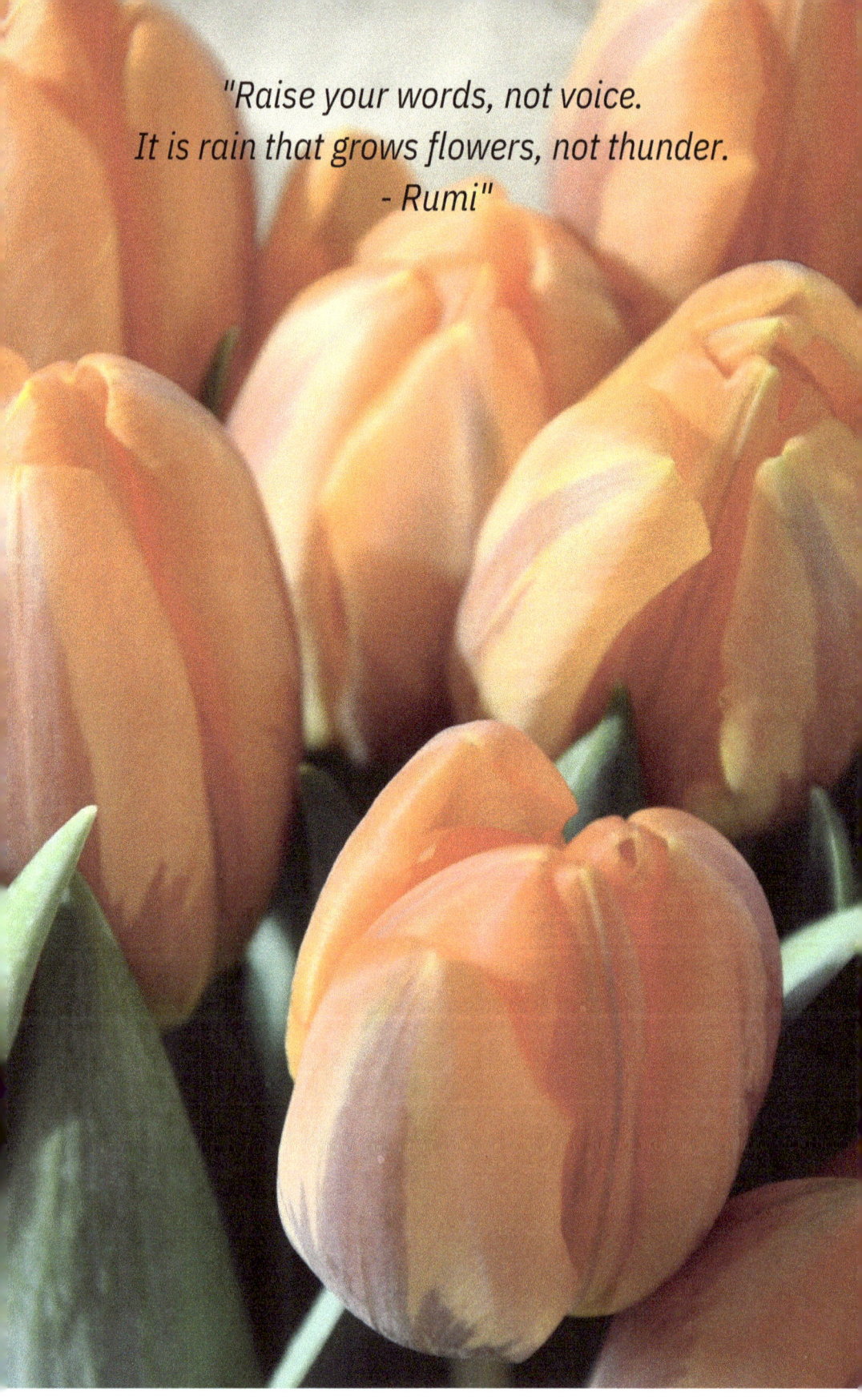

I CELEBRATE THANKSGIVING EVERY DAY. HOW ABOUT YOU?

I AM GRATEFUL FOR...

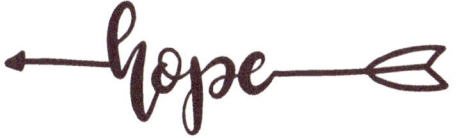

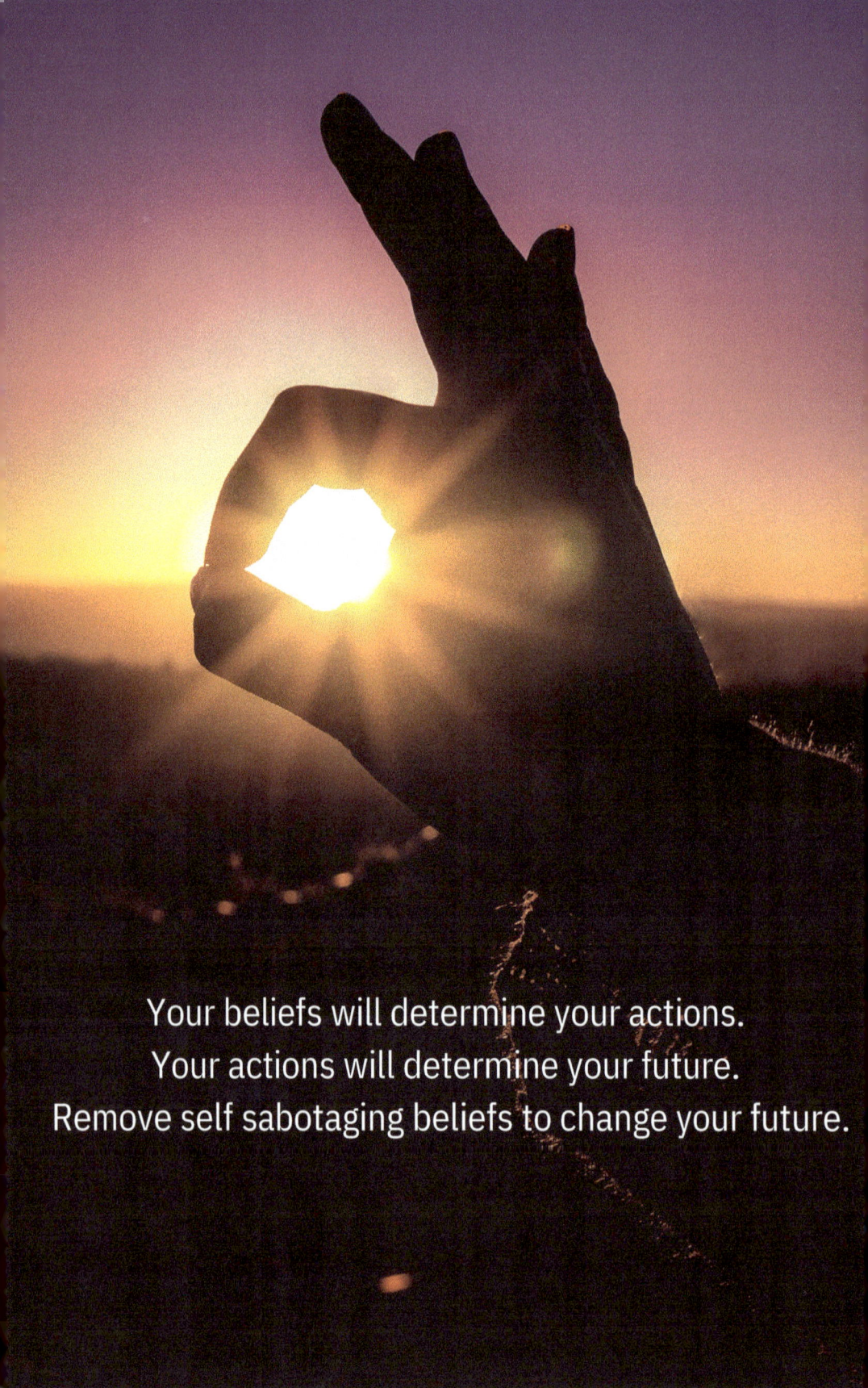

THANK YOU WITH A SMILE WILL OPEN DOORS TO ALL POSSIBLITIES."

I AM GRATEFUL FOR...

hope

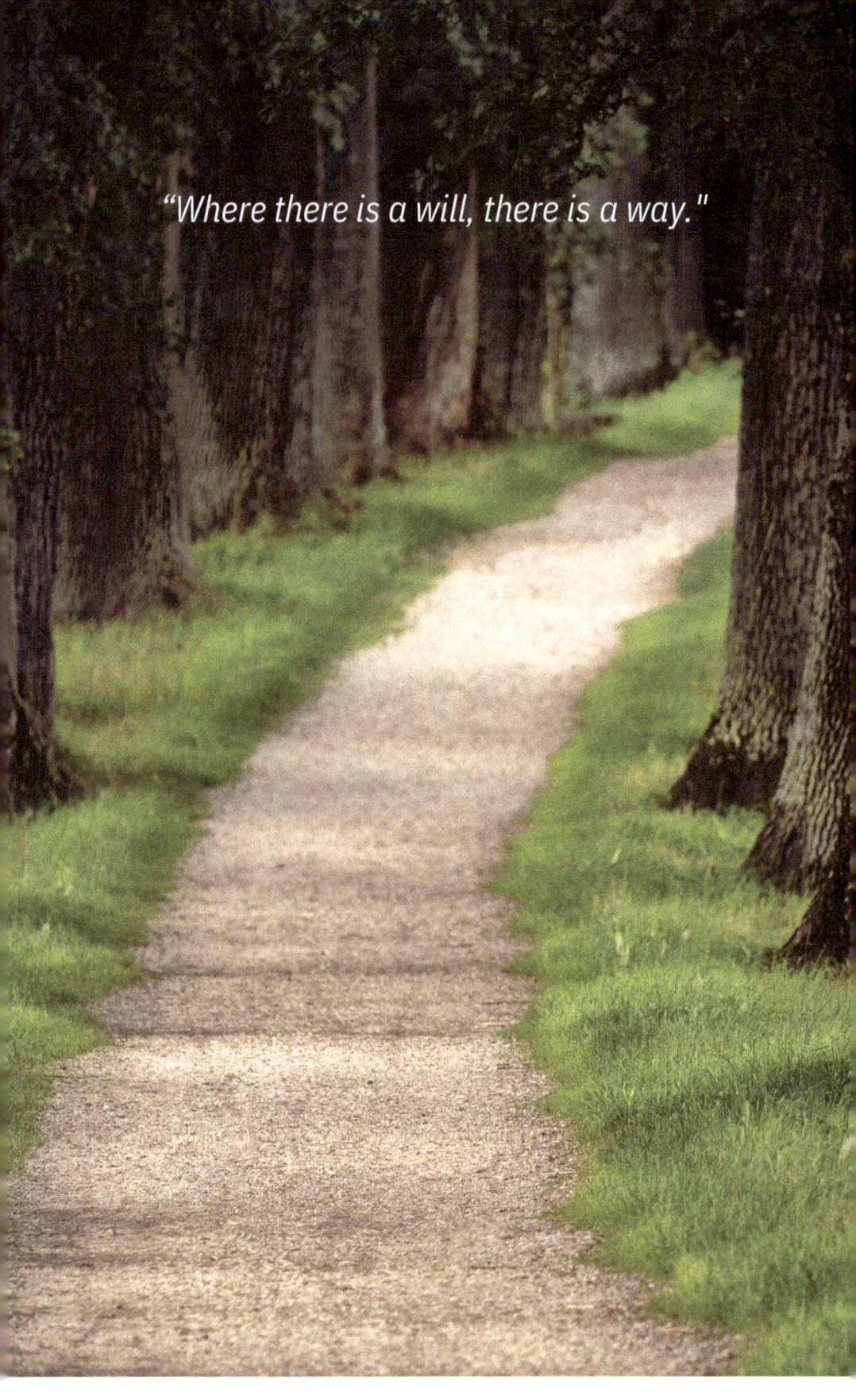

COUNT YOUR BLESSINGS EVERY MORNING AND YOUR DAY WILL BE MIRACULOUS.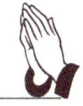

I AM GRATEFUL FOR...

hope

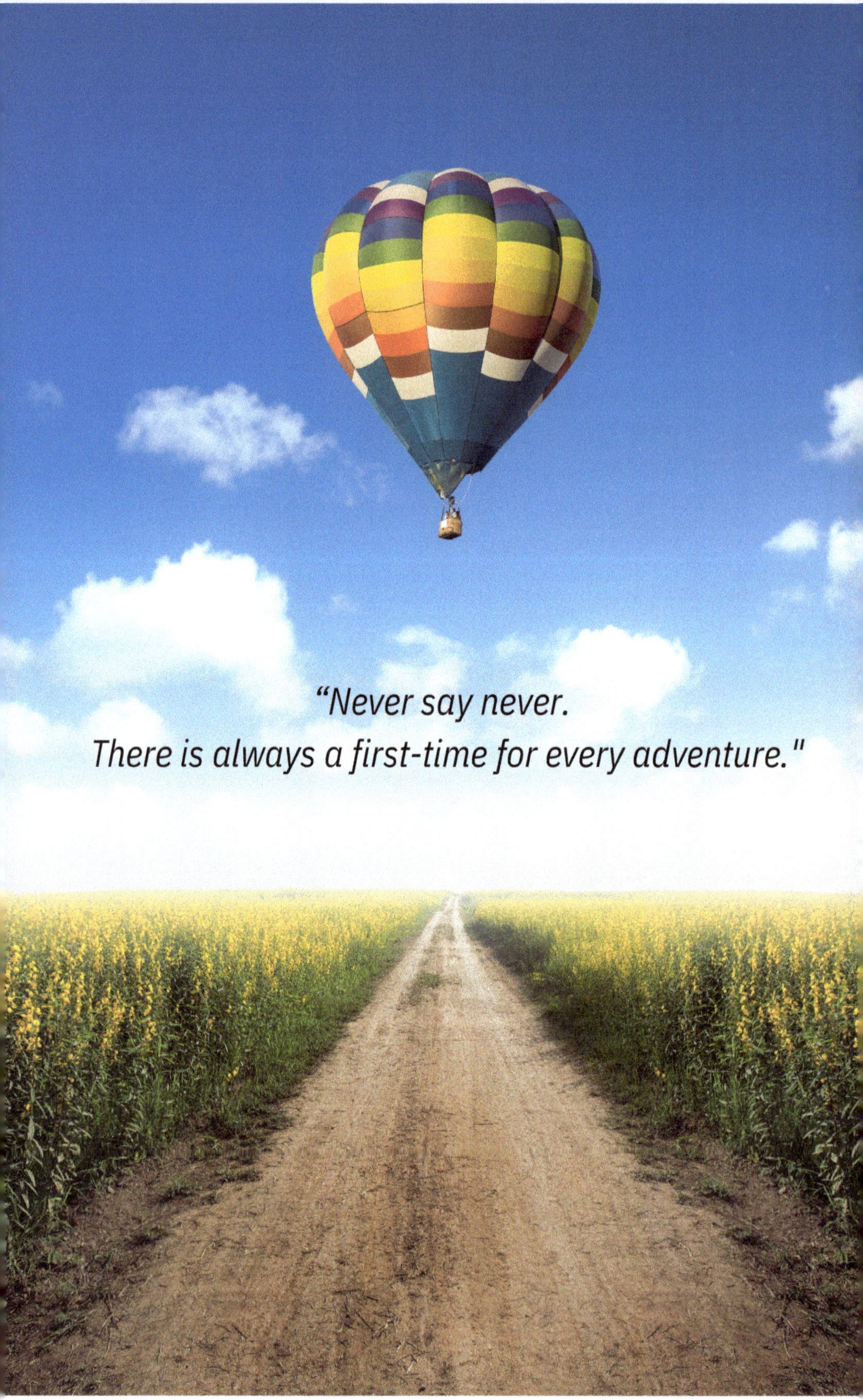

"Never say never.
There is always a first-time for every adventure."

AN ATTITUDE OF GRATITUDE IS LIKE A CUP OF HOT CHOCOLATE ON A COLD WINTER DAY.

I AM GRATEFUL FOR...

hope

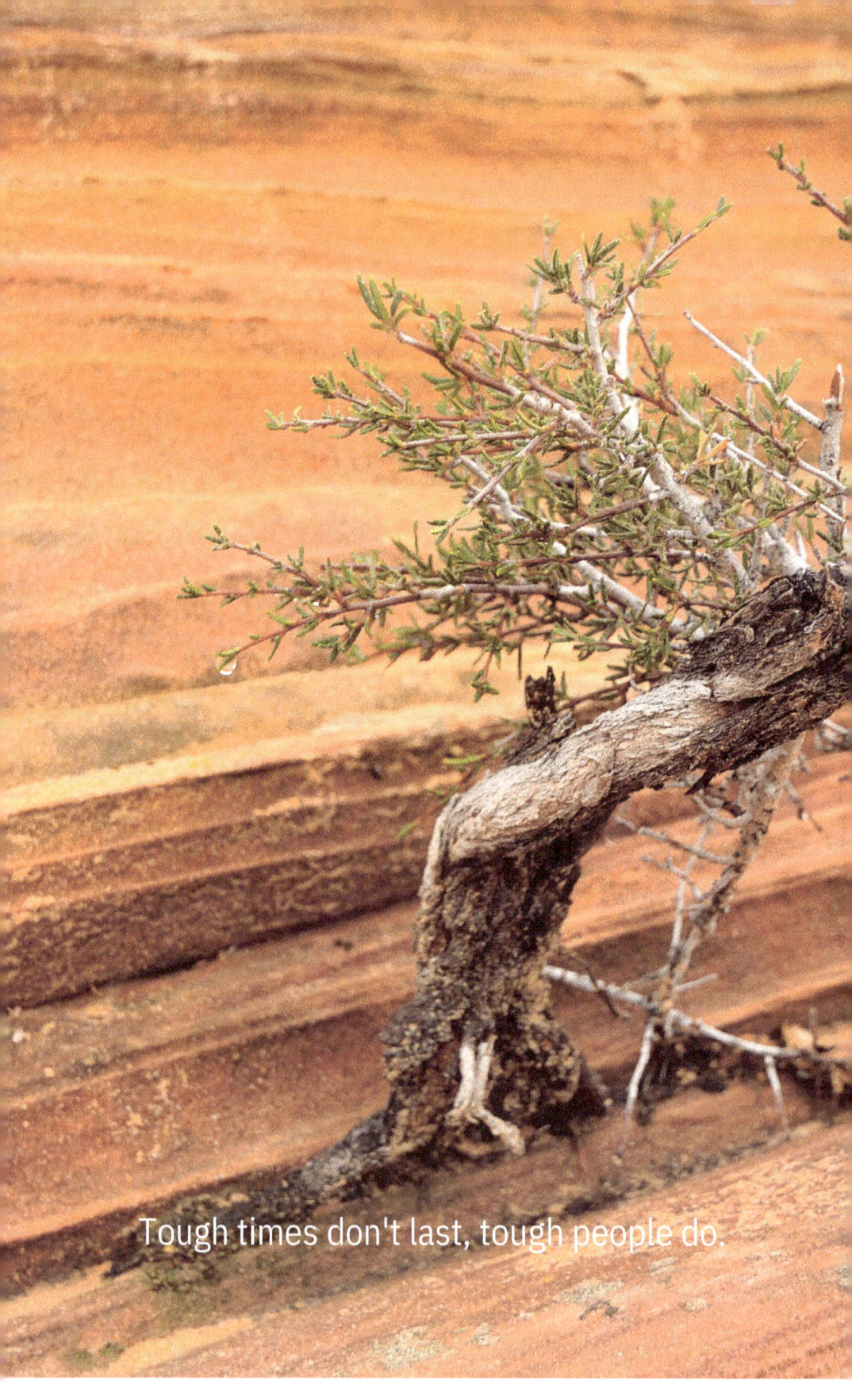

A PERSON WHO TREATS CRUMBS LIKE A FEAST EVENTUALLY GETS A FEAST.

I AM GRATEFUL FOR...

hope

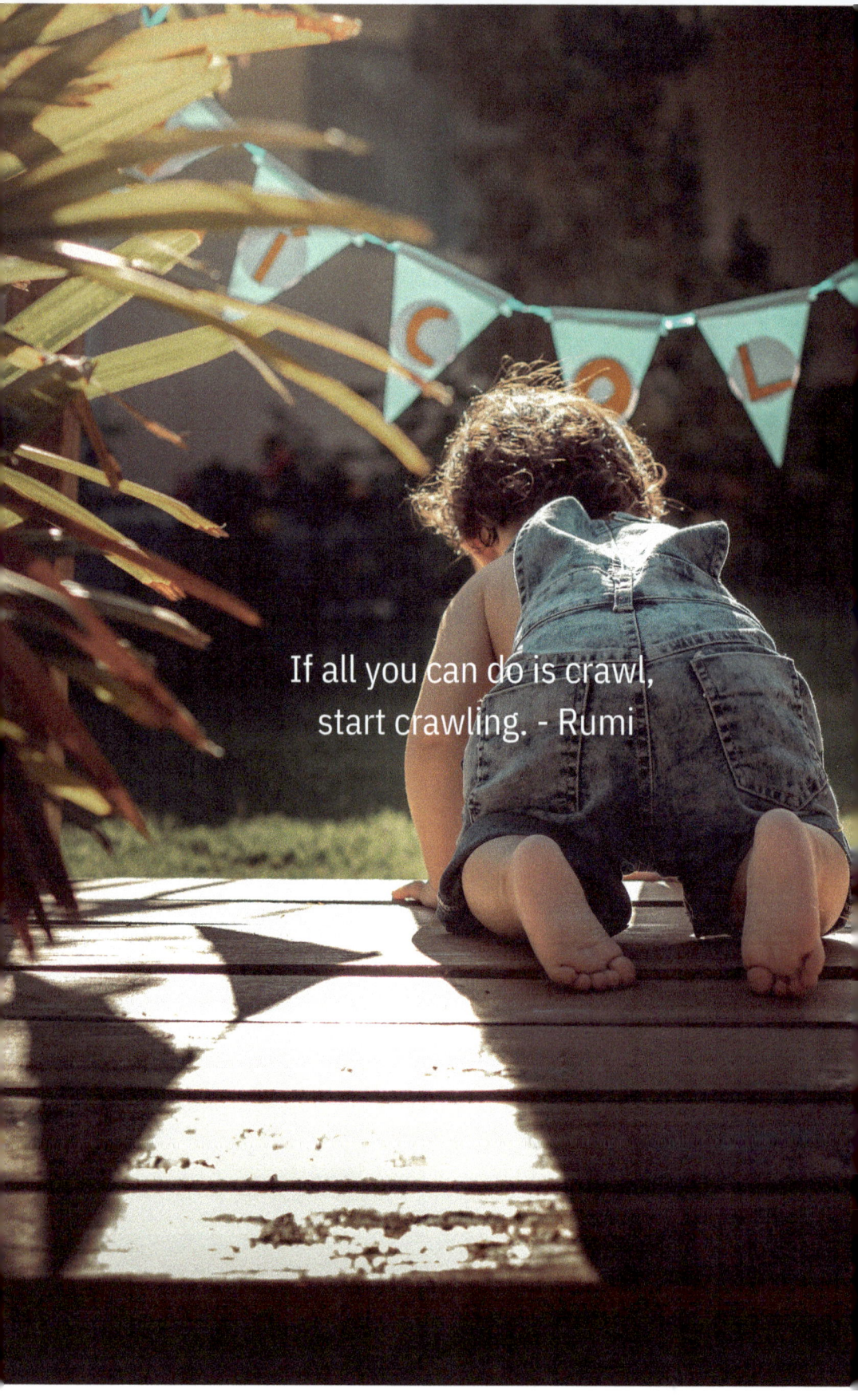

AN ATTITUDE OF GRATITUDE WILL BRING JOY TO A HEAVY HEART.

I AM GRATEFUL FOR...

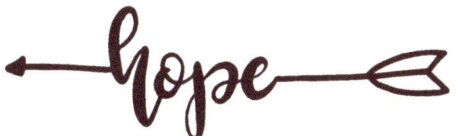

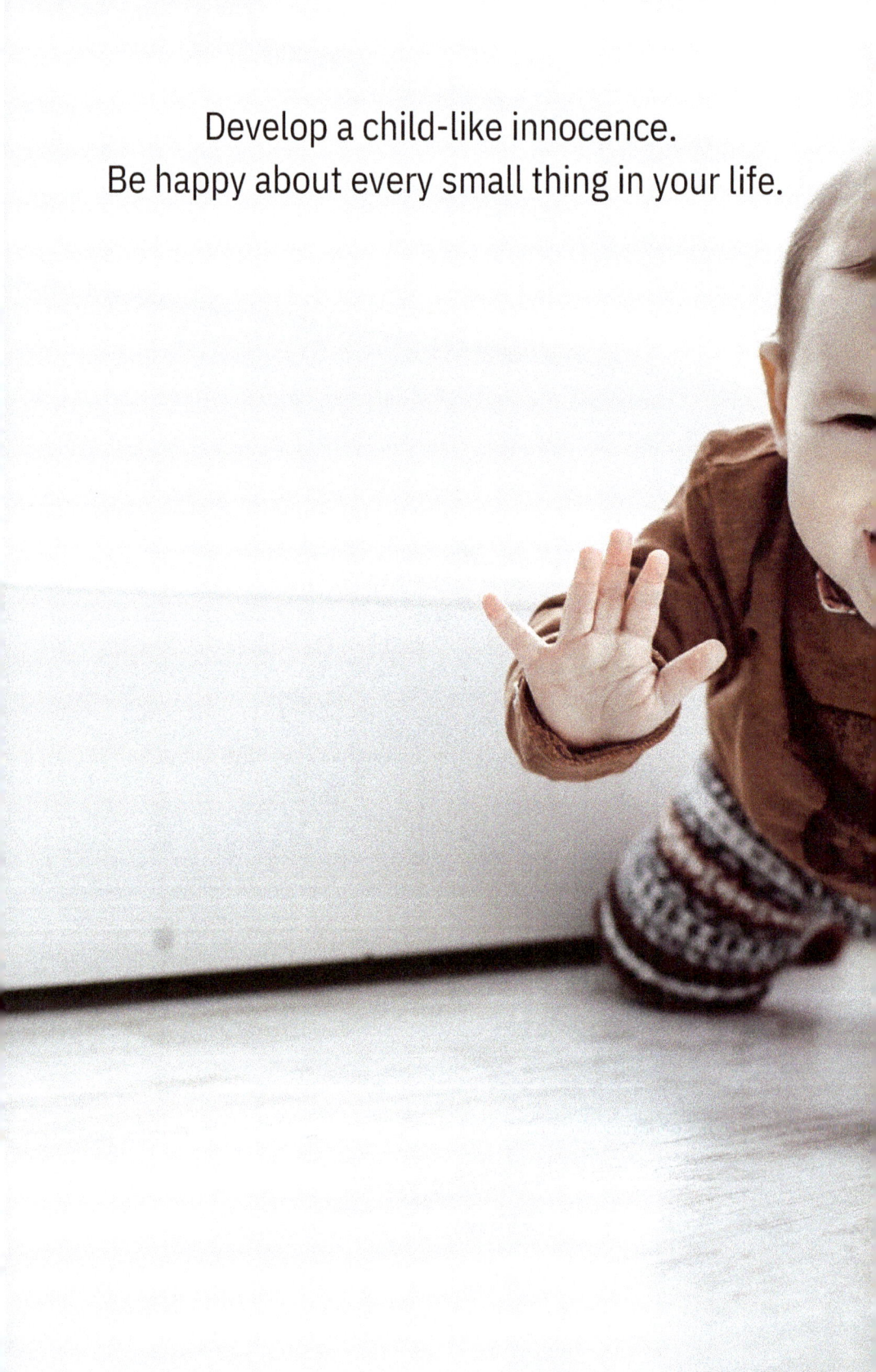

Develop a child-like innocence.
Be happy about every small thing in your life.

HAPPINESS IS NOT A DESTINATION. IT IS A JOURNEY. BE THANKFUL FOR EVERY STEP YOU TAKE.

I AM GRATEFUL FOR...

hope

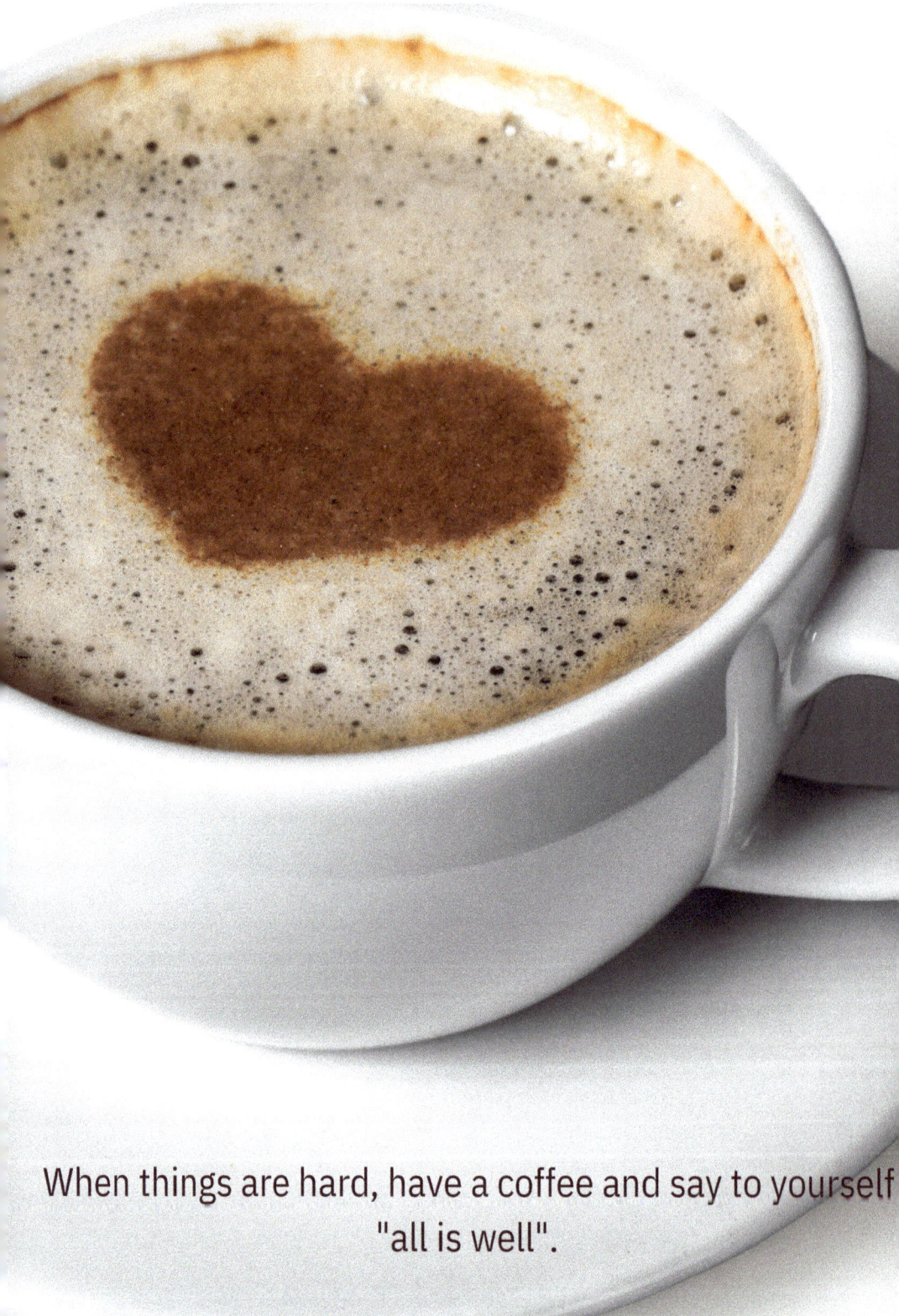

www.ingramcontent.com/pod-product-compliance
Lightning Source LLC
Chambersburg PA
CBHW040413070526
44119CB00139B/204